Public Health and Cold War Politics in Asia

Bu and her contributors illustrate the complexity of tensions and negotiations in the development of different types of public health systems in Asia during the early Cold War.

Competing models of development with different political ideologies and economic enterprises increasingly influenced Asian countries in their efforts to build modern nations after World War II. Looking at examples from China, Japan, South and North Korea, India, and Indonesia, the contributors to this volume look at how a range of Asian countries handled this postcolonial challenge. Health became a pivotal area that sustained the political discourse of differentiating one type of society from the other and promoting each system's advantages over the other's during the Cold War. Central to the discourse of a just society and the well-being of citizens was the promotion of public health and welfare for the people. The right to health was considered a fundamental human right as well as an essential social justice. A healthy population was also a prerequisite for national economic prosperity. Public health in postwar Asia was, therefore, a sociopolitical matter as well as a concern for the well-being of individuals. The health of the people demonstrated the advancement of a nation and provided the insurance for economic productivity and national prosperity.

An essential read for historians and policymakers of public health and historians of Asia during the Cold War.

Liping Bu is Reid-Knox Chair Professor and Chair of the History Department at Alma College, USA.

The Cold War in Asia
Series Editor: Professor Malcolm H. Murfett

A series of books that both explores and addresses some of the more important questions raised by the Cold War in Asia. This series isn't confined to single country studies alone, but welcomes contributions from research scholars who are tackling comparative issues within Asia during the time of the Cold War. Quality is our goal and this series reflects this objective by catering for work drawn from a number of disciplines.

If you work in the broad field of Cold War studies don't hesitate to get in touch with the series editor Professor Malcolm Murfett at King's College London (malcolm.murfett@kcl.ac.uk). Books, both single authored and edited manuscripts, should preferably be within the 60,000–100,000-word range, although we are also interested in shorter studies (25,000–50,000 words) that focus on elements of the Cold War struggle in Asia.

If you are working on a project that seems to fit these guidelines, please send a detailed proposal to the series editor. Every proposal will, of course, be subject to strict peer review. If the proposal is supported by experts in the field, it will be our aim to begin publishing the next volumes of this series within a year to eighteen months of the issuing of a contract to the author.

We look forward to hearing from you.

Science, Technology and the Cultural Cold War in Asia
From Atoms for Peace to Space Flight
Yuka Moriguchi Tsuchiya

Japan's Threat Perception during the Cold War
Balancing Threats and Vulnerabilities
Eitan Oren

The Barter Economy of the Khmer Rouge Labor Camps
Scott Pribble

Public Health and Cold War Politics in Asia
Edited by Liping Bu

For more information about this series, please visit: www.routledge.com/The-Cold-War-in-Asia/book-series/CWA

Public Health and Cold War Politics in Asia

Edited by Liping Bu

Routledge
Taylor & Francis Group

LONDON AND NEW YORK

First published 2024
by Routledge
4 Park Square, Milton Park, Abingdon, Oxon, OX14 4RN

and by Routledge
605 Third Avenue, New York, NY 10158

Routledge is an imprint of the Taylor & Francis Group, an informa business

British Library Cataloguing-in-Publication Data
A catalogue record for this book is available from the British Library

ISBN: 978-1-032-33092-1 (hbk)
ISBN: 978-1-032-33093-8 (pbk)
ISBN: 978-1-003-31816-3 (ebk)

DOI: 10.4324/9781003318163

Typeset in Galliard
by SPi Technologies India Pvt Ltd (Straive)

Contents

Contributors

Liping Bu is Reid-Knox Chair Professor and Chair of the History Department at Alma College, Michigan, USA. She has published numerous articles and books on public health, international education and cultural relations. Her books on public health include *Science, Public Health, and the State in Modern Asia* (2012); *Public Health and National Reconstruction in Post-War Asia* (2014); and *Public Health and the Modernization of China, 1865–2015* (2017).

Junho Jung is a Researcher at the Korean Research Institute of Science, Technology and Civilization, Jeonbuk National University, South Korea. He has numerous publications, including "Creating the Red Health Warrior: Ideological Struggle in North Korea's Health Care Sector, 1956–1961," *The Korean Journal for the History of Science* 40, no. 3 (2018) and "It All Started from Worms": Korea-Japan Parasite Control Cooperation and Asian Network, 1960s–1980s," *Korean Journal of Medical History* 27, no. 1 (2018). His research focuses on the transnationality of parasitology and parasite control programs in East Asia.

Park Yunjae is a Professor in the History Department at Kyung Hee University, and Director of HK+ Institute of Integrated Medical Humanities, Seoul, South Korea. He has numerous publications on medicine and health in colonial and modern Korea, including *The Origin of Korean Modern Medical System (Korean)* (2005) and *Modern History of Medicine in Korea (Korean)* (2021).

Shirish N. Kavadi is an independent researcher and a Visiting Professor in Political Science at Symbiosis International University, Pune, Maharashtra, India. His numerous publications include "Rockefeller Public Health in Colonial India," in *Histories of Medicine and Healing in the Indian Ocean World* (2016); "Medicine, Philanthropy and Nationhood: Tensions of Different Visions in India," in *Public Health and National Reconstruction in Post-War Asia* (2015); and "A Fractured Democracy: A Historical Overview of 'Science and Scholarship', Democratic Culture and the State in India," *Indian Philosophical Quarterly* 47 (2020).

Vivek Neelakantan is an independent historian of medicine and a Brocher Visiting Fellow. He has numerous publications, including *Science, Public Health and Nation-Building in Soekarno-Era Indonesia* (2017) and *The Geopolitics of Health in South and Southeast Asia: Perspectives from the Cold War to Covid-19* (2023). His research has been featured in leading international journals such as *ISIS Current Bibliography, Wellcome Open Research, Bijdragen tot de Taal-, Land-en Volkenkunde,* and *Southeast Asian Studies.* His current research investigates the origins of primary healthcare in Southeast Asia from a transnational perspective.

Takakazu Yamagishi is Director of the Center for International Affairs and a Professor on the Faculty of Global Liberal Studies at Nanzan University, Japan. He has extensive publications on public health, including *War and Health Insurance Policy in Japan and the United States: World War II to Postwar Reconstruction* (2011); *A History of American Health Care: The 20th Century Experience and Obamacare* (2014); and *Health Insurance Politics in Japan: Policy Development, the Government, and the Japan Medical Association* (2022).

Introduction*
Competing Models and Different Paths to Public Health

Liping Bu

Health policies and programs of the newly established governments in post–World War II (WWII) Asia aligned with their political visions and ideas of modernization and national development. Many Asian countries were directly affected by the rivalry between the United States and the Soviet Union in the emerging Cold War when they embarked on national reconstruction. The increasing tensions between the two superpowers complicated the process of nation-building and health construction, as the United States and the Soviet Union each promoted their own political ideologies and national development models as the order of the world. They influenced the postwar governments via political support, economic and military aid, and financial and professional assistance. The Cold War shaped and even polarized the directions of national development and health construction in various Asian countries as they proceeded with postwar recovery and reconstruction. This book uses six countries—China, Japan, North Korea, South Korea, India and Indonesia—as examples to examine how Cold War politics influenced health development when competing models and ideologies were promoted for the paths to public health.

World War II, the most devastating conflict that took more than 50 million people's lives, turned out to be a pivotal time of fundamental transition from foreign dominance to national independence in many Asian countries. During the war, anti-colonial groups joined the Allies to fight against fascist aggressions and colonial rule. Wartime promotion of democracy and freedom strengthened the aspirations of national liberation from foreign domination. The victory of WWII bolstered the hopes of colonized people to seek national independence and better lives. When the aggressors of Japan, Germany and Italy were defeated at the end of the war, old European colonial powers were also substantially weakened in the world. In Asia, WWII not only defeated Japan and ended its colonial empire but also precipitated the dissolution of the

* This book is indebted to Professor Shin Dongwon, who introduced the Korean scholars as chapter authors on South and North Korea. Thanks to Professor Shin Dongwon for sharing his recent research and publications and to Kyuri Kim for sharing her research presented at the 15th International Conference on the History of Science in East Asia.

DOI: 10.4324/9781003318163-1

British, the French, the American and the Dutch colonial rule. Full-scale decolonization movements and revolution swept across Asia, which led to the national independence of numerous countries from Western colonial powers in the wake of WWII. The new sovereign states set in motion a new process of modernization and national development.

National independence and revolution created a brand-new national identity. The sovereign states envisioned ambitious plans to transform their societies into strong modern nations with social improvement and economic prosperity. They promoted new political ideologies and patriotic feelings while creating new social and political institutions to implement national programs. In the state propagation of national prosperity and social justice, public health and the well-being of the people constituted a central promise of a better society. Good health was essential for people to live a happy and productive life. Public health was considered indispensable in the modern development of social justice, economic prosperity and a better life for the people. Furthermore, national economic prosperity relied on the productivity of a healthy population. An unhealthy population would not only drain the valuable resources of reconstruction but also result in the loss of productivity of workers. In the international community, a nation's health was an important gauge of its overall advancement. Hence, public health was a sociopolitical matter of the nation as much as a concern about the well-being of the people. Public health was an important and major component of modernization in both improving people's lives and securing national development.

Competing Models and Different Paths

The United States and the Soviet Union each influenced other countries with offers of economic and technical aid to promote their models of national development and modernization.[1] Advocates for the American model projected that a liberal capitalist system based on free market and private enterprises along with political democracy was the universal trajectory of socioeconomic development in the world.[2] The Soviet model promoted state planning of socioeconomic development, with emphasis on the equality of people to show the superiority of the socialist system.[3] The competing models of modernization significantly influenced the health policies of Asian nations when they engaged different political ideologies to underline the visions of national development amidst the Cold War politics of international relations. Immediately after WWII, the United States occupied and ruled Japan and South Korea. It provided the framework of postwar development for both countries before it ended the military rule in Japan in 1952 and in South Korea in 1948. When the United States defined the Cold War policy apparatus via the Truman Doctrine, the National Security Act and the formation of NATO between 1947 and 1949, the ruling policies in Japan and South Korea also took a drastic turn to anti-communist ideology.[4] In the meantime, the Soviet Union controlled North Korea after WWII and influenced the formation of the North Korean government. China fought a civil war between 1946 and 1949, with the Communists defeating the Nationalists. When the Communist-led revolution created the People's Republic of China on the mainland in 1949, the Nationalists retreated to Taiwan with the support of the United States.[5] The Soviet Union offered political support and economic aid to the People's Republic of China and North Korea and formed close relations. Both China and North Korea followed the Soviet model of state planning to carry out a socialist transformation of their societies. The newly independent countries from European empires, such as India and Indonesia, each hammered out their own visions of national development with strong decolonization orientation. They tried to stay neutral in the new international environment of Cold War politics and ideological rivalry. They championed the policy of independence by leading the Non-Aligned Movement as a third way of international relations.[6] Political neutrality to the two superpowers' hegemony, however, proved vulnerable and unsustainable under the pressure of foreign assistance and international aid. Studies show that their postwar reconstruction programs became negotiations between the preference of national priorities and the interference of superpowers.[7]

The United States, with its global economic dominance and influence, overshadowed the Soviet Union in extending technical, economic, and military aid as means to win political prestige and alliance. The Truman administration initiated the use of American technical know-how to win the competition. Truman's "Point Four" program called for "making the benefits of our scientific advances and industrial progress available for the improvement and growth of under-developed areas."[8] The Point Four program mobilized American universities, industries and philanthropic foundations to provide professional expertise and personnel, as well as technical and financial resources, for American international programs. The strategy of sharing American technical know-how and scientific advances proved an enormous soft power of the United States in the Cold War world.[9] A plethora of economic and technical aid programs were carried out overseas in the realms of public health, education, agriculture, industrial development, and military support. Numerous United States government agencies, such as the Mutual Security Agency, the Economic Cooperation Administration, and International Cooperation Administration (ICA, which became the United States Agency for International Development, USAID, in 1961) oversaw programs from public health to economic development and military cooperation in many countries. In the realm of health and medicine, international organizations—the World Health Organization (WHO) and the United Nations agencies—as well as American philanthropies of the Rockefeller Foundation (RF) played significant roles, often in collaboration and cooperation with American overseas programs. Health historian Marcos Cueto points out that international health became an important tool of foreign policy during the Cold War.[10] The professional guidance and financial assistance of international and transnational organizations helped shape the design of public health and health systems of different countries with less overt Cold War politicization.

National interests and local political and economic conditions, however, often defined the delivery of health programs. National initiatives and local creative measures constantly negotiated national preferences with external influence in the interactions with international organizations and the two superpowers. National priorities of development decided whether the government would commit resources to health construction and improvement of healthcare, even though the rivalry between the United States and the Soviet Union affected the direction of development in various Asian countries. In the everyday politics of the Cold War, public health became the arena where political discourse promoted the values and differentiations of one system over the other in the dichotomy of freedom and democracy vs. state planning and equality of people.

Asian nations strove for national advancement with national health construction as they all faced the challenges of widespread diseases and serious health problems after the war. Epidemics, such as cholera, tuberculosis, smallpox, dysentery, yaws, malaria and leprosy, devastated many countries. From the newly independent countries of Korea, India and Indonesia to the revolutionary China and the American-occupied Japan, epidemic diseases ran rampant. Modern medical innovations offered great expectations in the treatment and prevention of diseases. The newly established governments were eager to use the latest available medical knowledge and technology in fighting diseases and improving health conditions. However, they lacked resources, manpower and technical expertise in combating diseases. Health personnel and facilities were in desperate need of updating and expansion. Moreover, the pressing issues of building a viable health system and effective public health programs were further complicated by war devastation, poverty, political instability and ethnic conflicts.

In the creation of health programs and medical research, Cold War politics and international economic aid influenced the strategies and policies of health development in different Asian countries. Competing models of national development with distinct ideological orientations for different economic systems increasingly defined Asian countries as following either the United States or the Soviet Union when the world fell into a bipolar order centered around the two superpowers. Health became a pivotal area where the Cold War political discourse differentiated one type of society from the other in promoting advantages of one system over the other. Between the socialist and the capitalist systems lay a type of hybrid that used both private and public services, purportedly neutral to the superpowers' rivalry for ideological dominance. National interests and policy priorities, based on local economic conditions and health infrastructure, appeared crucial in the negotiations with the powers of international aid for the national agenda of health construction. The political ideologies and policy priorities of each Asian country, coupled with local health infrastructure and socioeconomic conditions, led to the different outcomes of national health systems and public health programs. Studies of the six countries in this book illustrate the different paths to national development and health construction during the Cold War.

The concepts of health and healthcare gained new meanings and understanding in Asian countries after WWII. In countries such as the People's Republic of China and the Democratic Republic of Korea, the concept of the people's health was promoted, with the state projecting the vision of universal free healthcare for the people as an important aspect of the socialist transformation of the society. The hallmark of the people's health was the state responsibility for people's health, which was hailed as the superiority and advantage of the socialist system over the capitalist system. Physicians and medical professionals, who used to be the social elite of the educated class, underwent reeducation to reform their old attitude and to learn to serve the people as health workers. Socialist values were promoted to treat people as equals and to work for the common good.

In Japan and South Korea, where American influence dominated, the concept of public health was promoted, with private enterprises operating health insurance programs. The Supreme Commander for the Allied Powers (SCAP) initially toyed with the idea of creating a national health system for Japan, but the idea was quickly abandoned when Cold War politics reoriented the policies with strong anti-communist ideology and rejected the role of government in healthcare. Japan's health construction continued with the existing infrastructure of health insurance programs that were built during wartime. After the American occupation ended in 1952, the Japanese government expanded health insurance programs and increased its role in the national health system toward universal healthcare. In South Korea, the concept of public health was also promoted. The government under Syngman Rhee relied on American and international aid for disease control and healthcare. After the military coup in 1961, the South Korean government attempted to address national health matters by introducing medical insurance acts in the 1960s but committed little national recourses to health construction. Only after South Korea's economy took a dramatic turn of growth in the 1970s did the government pay attention to the improvement of public health by following the Japanese model of health insurance. In both Japan and South Korea, the health insurance system was promoted as freedom of choice in the Cold War political discourse to contrast with socialist state planning. Great variations of payment and benefits existed in the different programs of health insurance. People's access to insurance programs depended on their status and profession in society. The free choice of health insurance programs worked well for the rich and powerful but not for the less fortunate majority. In order to address the issues of affordability and accessibility, the Japanese and South Korean governments subsidized health insurance programs. As a result, the role of the state increased significantly in healthcare.

India and Indonesia, after their independence, both promoted health as a fundamental right of the people, with the operation of public and private health services. The concept of health as a human right was promoted in the decolonization discourse of national development. The central government made health policies, while the local governments were responsible for the delivery of health programs and services. India's constitution specified that the national government was responsible to ensure the "right to health" for all people, regardless of their status, and that each state was to provide healthcare services for the people. In Indonesia, the government made public health an important part of nation-building. It created a public health system with nationalized hospitals and health facilities but allowed physicians to keep their private practice on the side. The national government in both India and Indonesia relied significantly on international aid and health assistance.

This book presents the latest research on public health in different Asian countries during the Cold War. Drawing on local archives and native language publications, the chapters examine the various aspects of national health construction that were complicated by Cold War politics. Their cutting-edge research and theoretical concepts offer fresh insights into the complexity of political calculations of economic aid and the connections between public health and economic growth. They analyze the tensions between national interests and international interference in the development of health programs. The studies of the six countries—China, Japan, North Korea, South Korea, India and Indonesia—highlight a comparative view of the approaches of health construction under different sociopolitical systems in Cold War Asia. The chapter authors investigate how public health was related to economic development and how different political systems viewed the role of public health in society. Their analysis of the different forces internal and external in shaping up public health programs illuminate how the competing ideologies and political values informed health policies that profoundly affected the everyday life of ordinary people. They also demonstrate that local health infrastructure, socioeconomic conditions and political aspirations were important factors that contributed to the development of health policies and programs.

The People's Health: China and North Korea

China and North Korea carried out a socialist transformation of their societies with extensive public health movements to build the people's health. The policies that defined the people's health emphasized expansion of health training programs and ideological reeducation of health professionals to serve the people. The policies emphasized prevention as the priority of epidemic disease control. The two countries differed in programs and practices in many areas because of factors such as different health conditions in each country, national policy preferences and the impact of international assistance. Health policies in both countries emphasized the people's health to demonstrate the state's responsibility and commitment to improving people's lives. The policies gained the support of the people for the government's national development agenda. A healthy population was essential in ensuring the manpower for national economic productivity as well as the well-being of individuals. The state made the construction of the people's health an integral part of the overall socioeconomic transformation of the society, with political mobilization of the people to participate in socialist nation-building. To change the society and the people, health work was integrated in the general political movement of criticizing the exploitations of capitalism and reeducating the people, including health professionals, about the socialist values of equality and the common good.

Both China and North Korea followed the Soviet model in their initial state planning of national recovery and socialist transformation. Soviet medical science and preventive methods influenced the health knowledge and work in China and North Korea, as discussed by the chapters in this book. However, they each developed, despite the Soviet influence, their own approaches and methods as well as policy orientations that were based on local knowledge, experience and conditions. In terms of external assistance, China received aid primarily from the Soviet Union only in the 1950s, while North Korea received assistance from a broader range of countries, including the Soviet Union, China and socialist Eastern European countries. In the late 1950s when tensions arose within the communist camp, particularly due to the increasing disagreements between China and the Soviet Union after the Soviet leader Nikita Khrushchev made a drastic policy shift, both China and North Korea began to emphasize self-reliance in national development. China's relations with the Soviet Union deteriorated further, which led to the end of Soviet aid and full-blown hostilities between the two countries by 1960. North Korea, while trying delicately to balance relations with China and the Soviet Union with aid from both countries, accomplished its own achievements with health campaigns and the Chollima Movement.

China

When the People's Republic of China was established in 1949, China finally gained peace with the end of decades-long devastating wars. The country, however, faced a collapsed economic and financial system, widespread poverty and rampant epidemic diseases. The new government, being the people's sovereignty, launched sanitation and health campaigns, and socioeconomic reforms immediately after it took power. Health campaigns aimed at combating twenty-some types of major epidemic diseases that had crippled the lives of millions of people and the economic activities of towns and villages. Moreover, China suffered severe shortages of medicine, health facilities and professional manpower. The government emphasized disease prevention as the first priority with political mobilization of the people to participate in the anti-disease campaigns. Traditional Chinese medicine, which was more accessible and affordable than Western biomedicine, was promoted in combination with the use of Western medicine. National health policy defined the people's health as the principle of health work, and healthcare was to serve the needs of the people, specifically that of workers, peasants and soldiers. Hospitals and clinics were nationalized and renamed the people's hospitals and clinics.

The success of the Communist-led revolution in establishing a new government in mainland China "alarmed" the United States at a time when the Cold War politics and policies were shaping up the United States' global outlook. The United States and China were allies during WWII. The United States was deeply involved in pushing for a coalition government in China after the war. It sent two missions to China in an attempt to bring the Nationalists and the Communists together to form a coalition government, with Patrick Hurley leading the mission in August-October 1945 and George Marshall leading the mission in December 1945–January 1946.[11] Both missions failed the colossal task of creating a coalition government in China. The United States ended up supporting the Nationalists against the Communists in the ensuing civil war. When the Communists defeated the Nationalists and founded the People's Republic of China (PRC), the United States was bitterly disappointed. In the United States, the Republicans blamed the Democrats for "the loss of China," as if China were a possession of the United States.[12] The United States used economic sanctions, military threats and the political pressure of international isolation to punish the PRC and prevent it from success. It denied the diplomatic recognition of the PRC government and continued the support of the Nationalists in Taiwan. In the meantime, the Soviet Union offered support to the PRC with economic aid and technical assistance. China and the Soviet Union signed the Sino-Soviet Treaty of Friendship, Alliance and Mutual Assistance in 1950.

The Soviet Union asserted a significant but short-term influence on China's socialist transformation in the 1950s. Learning from the Soviet Union became the slogan in China when the country embarked on national reconstruction. Soviet science, particularly Pavlov's theories, and health knowledge were promoted in health and medical studies and research, reorienting Chinese medical education and medical epidemiology. Soviet methods of preventive medicine were introduced and applied to Chinese health programs and anti-disease campaigns. One of the successful examples of Soviet influence was the concept of using prevention centers to direct local health communication and disease control. China followed the Soviet model in establishing the Health and Epidemic Prevention Station as the center to lead disease prevention in every city district, rural county and town. The station was a government health agency that provided comprehensive disease prevention measures, immunization and health education and coordinated local health research and campaigns. The local health and epidemic prevention stations eventually formed a national network of disease prevention administration under the Ministry of Health. A holistic social approach to disease prevention was carried out along with disseminating health information and extensive vaccination.[13]

China's disease prevention was integrated in the overall socioeconomic development of the society. It was an important endeavor to modernize China into a healthy and strong country since the early twentieth century.[14]

The PRC's state planning of national economic growth and social transformation included programs of disease control and eradication to improve people's health and promote economic production. The comprehensive social approach to disease prevention and health improvement was manifested in the nationwide sanitation and hygiene campaigns whereby people were mobilized to actively combat diseases. Health workers educated people about diseases and healthy behavior with visual materials to popularize scientific knowledge and to change people's old views and attitudes.[15] The campaigns brought new energies into health work that united people to build a better society. Grassroots health campaigns purported to turn the masses into an active force of disease prevention rather than being marginalized as passive recipients of medical treatment. This change in people's role in health work echoed the political discourse that the people were the master of their own society. Community cooperation and collaboration during the health campaigns proved positive in disease control, such as the prevention of malaria, schistosomiasis, and tuberculosis.

Health policies emphasized the building of basic-level health infrastructure and the expansion of health training programs at all levels in order to meet the needs of health services. Health clinics and centers in urban cities and rural towns formed a national infrastructure of primary healthcare. Urban district health centers were connected with city hospitals and municipal health institutions, while rural health institutions consisted of a three-tiered network of county hospitals, rural town hospitals and village health stations. Women's and children's hospitals were established with the expansion of training new midwives and assistant nurses as well as the retraining of nearly one million old-style midwives.[16] The central government promulgated free medical services to state workers and members of political parties and organizations in 1952, while rural collectives formed medical cooperatives in the 1950s.

Relations with the Soviet Union began to deteriorate in the late 1950s after Nikita Khrushchev started the de-Stalinist movement and promoted a new international policy of peaceful coexistence with the West. Khrushchev's change of policies caused serious discords among communist countries, with China becoming a leading critic of Khrushchev.[17] China began to shift toward more self-reliance in economic development. The Great Leap Forward was launched in 1958 to accelerate industrial and agricultural growth along with health reconstruction and social transformation. People's communes were speedily established in the rural agricultural sector, whereas industries were pushed to expand production without solid technical foundations. Health construction underwent major changes as well. Within the people's commune system, commune-sponsored collective medical cooperatives were formed to provide healthcare for farmers and rural population. Rural medical cooperatives were developed in parallel to the state-sponsored medical care for state employees in cities. However, the need for health services was enormous in rural China, where more than 80 percent of the Chinese population lived. City hospitals sent mobile teams of doctors to rural communes to help with medical treatment and training, but they were not able to meet the needs. To tackle the problem, the Health Ministry began short-term education programs to train large numbers of part-time health workers in the communes. The trainees were selected from rural youth who were farmers and they would return to their communities to serve their fellow villagers after training. The trainees learned rudimentary knowledge of Chinese and Western medicine and gained a good command of skills in disease prevention. The part-time rural health workers worked with farmers in the farming fields. They were called "barefoot doctors," a revolutionary endearment during the Cultural Revolution. In 1975, more than five million barefoot doctors were working in rural communes, where health institutions and hospital beds had increased to 60 percent of national totals.[18]

China took a road of its own in health construction after relations with the Soviet Union became hostile. Its economy developed with a dual structure of state and collective enterprises, where the agricultural sector and some local businesses were defined as collective enterprises in contrast to state enterprises. As the government-financed universal healthcare was integrated into the economic system, a parallel of state and collective health programs developed in the 1960s and 1970s that tied directly with the types of enterprises people worked at. State health programs had better benefits than collective health programs.

Liping Bu's chapter examines the Soviet aid to and American isolation of China when the country embarked on postwar reconstruction and socialist transformation. Chinese health policies defined the people's health with emphasis on building basic-level healthcare services for the general population. Learning from the Soviet Union was the slogan of national development when the United States treated the PRC with hostility. The chapter analyzes the tensions of the Cold War and its impact on health policies and programs in China, along with various political and social movements. In the discussion of the diverse programs of urban and rural healthcare, the study explores the political and social meanings of the people's health. The barefoot doctors and the rural medical cooperatives constituted the most significant development of health infrastructure in socialist China. The research on the people's health shows that during the high time of the Cold War when relations with the Soviet Union deteriorated and tensions with the United States continued, China carved out an independent road of socialist development with its own unique experience and practice often engulfed in radical political movements.

North Korea

North Korea promoted the people's health with free universal healthcare. It developed the health system based on local health conditions, international assistance and national policy preferences. When WWII ended the Japanese colonial rule, the sovereignty of Korea was restored. To the Korean people, WWII was the national liberation war. Unfortunately, the Korean Peninsula was divided into two at the 38th parallel at the end of the war, with the United States occupying the South and the Soviet Union the North. Two radically different political systems were thereafter established on the peninsula. In the emerging Cold War, South Korea became an ally of the United States, whereas North Korea an ally of the Soviet Union. When the Korean War broke out in 1950, the peninsula became the location of direct confrontation between the two rival sides of the Cold War, making East Asia a zone of two hostile camps.

In the realm of health and healthcare, both South and North Korea witnessed a fundamental change of the concept of health, shifting from Japanese colonial hygiene to post-liberation public health. Korean medical historian Shin Dong-won defines this conceptual change as a transformation from the age of "Wisang" (hygiene) to the era of "Pogŏn" (public health).[19] A new understanding of health developed in terms of the different operations of public health in North and South Korea. In North Korea, the government advocated the people's health, with an emphasis on building health facilities to deliver free health services to the general population. The Bureau of Public Health was established in October 1945, and it promoted the people's health to improve people's lives and to eradicate the legacy of Japanese coercive hygiene. Influenced by the Soviet Union, North Korea envisioned the building of a socialist society and the construction of people's healthcare. In South Korea, the concept of public health was promoted as the U.S. military government abolished the Japanese colonial Hygiene Department and established a Ministry of Health and Welfare. American ideas and practices were introduced to South Korea. As the North and the South followed different ideologies of nation-building, the political discourse of health in South Korea touted private healthcare and free citizenship, whereas the political promotion of health in North Korea advocated state-sponsored free healthcare and equality of the people.

North Korea passed the General Free Healthcare Act in 1950. Health policies emphasized epidemic prevention and disinfection as the first priority. Authorities launched large-scale hygiene education campaigns with the participation of workers and farmers. Health campaigns taught people basic hygienic knowledge and healthy behavior, such as not to eat raw vegetables or meat. As in China, the North Korean government coordinated hygiene campaigns in urban and rural areas with multiple sectors, such as transportation, education and agriculture, to work with the Bureau of Public Health.

In the early stage of socialist healthcare, national people's hospitals lowered drug prices and doctors' fees to make health services and treatment accessible to more people. Government policy prioritized to "expand the number of national hospitals, to eradicate epidemics, and to provide poor people with free medical care."[20] The government was eager to show a rapid increase of hospitals and clinics to fundamentally improve the health of the people. In rural areas, where the majority of people lived with no modern medical facilities, the government established branches of hospitals and circulated doctors throughout villages. These efforts were assisted by aid from the Soviet Union and China, as well as medical teams from socialist Eastern European countries when North Korea lacked health professionals.[21]

The transformation of health emphasized socialist education of health professionals, in which they criticized doctors as being unkind and arrogant toward ordinary people during the Japanese colonial rule. Health professionals, especially intellectual medical doctors, were reeducated to serve the people wholeheartedly in daily practice. They were expected to become ideologically superior and more progressive than the medical personnel in capitalist societies like the United States and South Korea. At the same time, North Korean authorities improved doctors' physical living conditions in terms of housing and wages. In the political mobilization to build a new people's Korea, officials denounced the colonial rule of Japanese imperialists for paying little attention to the health needs of Korean people when epidemic diseases of cholera, smallpox and typhus ran rampant.[22]

The North Korean government expanded the free healthcare system to all people in 1953 after the Korean War. With assistance from the Soviet Union and China, North Korea experienced an era of economic recovery and rapid industrialization from the 1950s through the 1970s. The improvement of health facilities and the overall health conditions for the people was a vital part of the economic recovery and security for the people. The government expanded the construction of health infrastructure by building health clinics in rural towns and villages, multiplying medical colleges and research projects, establishing children's hospitals and daycare centers, and training daycare workers. When tensions increased between China and the Soviet Union in the late 1950s, North Korea launched the Chollima Movement, as China did with the Great Leap Forward, to mobilize people to work harder for the country with the socialist drive. The movement was an attempt to speed up industrialization and economic prosperity with less dependence on foreign aid.

North Korea began to encourage the people to use traditional medicine in the late 1950s as an alternative to biomedicine in order to meet the needs for medical and preventive drugs. The shift to the usage of traditional medicine was influenced by China's success in the use of traditional medicine.[23] Some researchers explained that China's medical support and exchange of health knowledge played a crucial role in North Korea's rediscovery of traditional medicine.[24] In particular, China's emphasis on the combination of Chinese and Western medicine and the successful experiments convinced North Korean leaders the appropriate use of traditional medicine. The use of traditional medicine fit well with North Korea's search for domestic resources to increase self-reliance, as there was a significant decrease in foreign aid from the late 1950s into the early 1960s.[25]

North Korea created a national health system that was financed and operated by the state. The government invested significantly in building health facilities and training health personnel to ensure the successful implementation of free healthcare and free education. A healthcare network of provincial, county and village was created. Doctors, based at village clinics, were "directly accountable for provision of primary care to a select block of houses in each community."[26] Healthcare at the primary level was a distinctive feature of North Korean health system, and the healthcare coverage was uniform across the nation. However, despite the uniform health coverage, resources were prioritized for the capital Pyeongyang and other major cities to build large hospitals with the best medical equipment and personnel. Rural areas and minor towns were generally equipped with dispensaries and small clinics. There were some cases in which the collectives used their own budget to build clinics while the central government covered the expenses of daily operation.[27]

The rapid expansion of healthcare infrastructure and personnel resulted in twenty times more hospital beds available per person in North Korea than in South Korea by 1970.[28] North Korea was able to achieve the expansion of healthcare services due to the economic growth in those decades with crucial support from China and the Soviet Union, as well as the medical aid teams of Eastern European countries.[29] The period from 1953 through the 1970s witnessed the fast growth of North Korean economy that significantly outpaced the gross national product per capita of South Korea. Free healthcare services and economic prosperity made people in North Korea feel better and superior to South Korea, where many people could not afford to have modern healthcare in the same period. By the 1980s, government sources reported that universal healthcare access had been achieved.[30]

Junho Jung studies the eradication of paragonimiasis in his chapter on North Korea's social change and disease control. The study illuminates the concept of public health as an ideology for the socialistic transformation of ecology and society. It examines the paragonimiasis epidemic as a serious cause of workforce crisis and a catalyst for North Korea's search for knowledge and effective methods to tackle the disease, along with political mobilization of health campaigns. The chapter analyzes the nature of North Korea's healthcare through the examination of how North Koreans responded to individual diseases that hindered their socialistic nation-building. Jung investigates the social characteristics of North Korea and the ecological environment that caused health problems and the loss of labor. His research shows that North Korea attempted a socialist transformation of the people as citizens as well as the entire ecosystem that formed the material basis of socialist life. Furthermore, the chapter illustrates how medical knowledge and practice were transferred and implemented in North Korea through the transnational and international networks brought about by the Cold War.

Private Health Insurance: Japan and South Korea

South Korea

South Korea was under the American military government from 1945 to 1948. Postwar conditions in South Korea were characterized by widespread unrest among the populace and rampant epidemic diseases of tuberculosis, typhus and cholera. The acute epidemic diseases posed significant challenges to the American military rule, whose first priority was to safeguard the protection of American troops and calm the social unrest. In tackling diseases and health problems, the American military government abolished the former Japanese colonial Bureau of Hygiene and established the Ministry of Health and Welfare. Corresponding health departments were also created in provinces to replace the Japanese colonial hygiene system. The American military government relied primarily on its military doctors and supplies to provide medical service and protection for the troops, as South Korea had few modern medical professionals. For the health needs of the public, the military government sought help from American private organizations such as the Rockefeller Foundation. The RF had a long history in Asia, where it had set up health stations and centers to control communicable diseases in several countries since the early 20th century.[31] Collaborating with the military government in South Korea, the RF built health centers in big cities of Seoul, Pusan and Chŏnju to conduct medical relief work, vaccination, health education and statistical collection. Each health center had a staff of a physician officer and a few nurses and assistants responsible for the work. The American military government promoted a free-market economy and relied on the private practice of Western biomedicine in the delivery of healthcare. The emphasis on private practice of medicine and capitalist-market healthcare further intensified the problems of the urban concentration of physicians, leaving rural villages with no doctors.[32] For poor Koreans who had little access to modern medicine, traditional medicine was the source of healing and treatment of diseases. At the end of the occupation in 1948, the American military government had made little progress in solving the political, economic and health problems in South Korea.[33]

American policies in South Korea shifted toward establishing an anti-communist Korea, with explicit anti-Soviet propaganda as an important policy objective.[34] The American Military Governor of Korea, Lieutenant General John Reed Hodge, claimed that free-market liberal ideology guaranteed individualism, creativity and freedom of expression in South Korea. He criticized North Korea's socialist approach to healthcare as the coercive execution of revolutionary decrees without citizens' voluntary consent.[35] Contrary to his remarks, South Koreans explicitly expressed their expectation of the government to provide healthcare. Political parties and medical professional organizations demanded state-sponsored medical care for the general population. The Korean Democratic Party called for equal opportunity of healthcare, the New Korean National Party supported public management of healthcare facilities, the Korean Independence Party demanded a nationwide establishment of people's healthcare facilities and the Nation-Founding Association argued for a comprehensive nationalization of healthcare.[36] The Korean Science Alliance even argued for a democratic reform of the healthcare system and the transformation of medical research in a democratic direction with a focus on preventative medicine.[37]

After the American military rule, the South Korean government continued the free-market policy of healthcare but decreased its commitment to public health. It abolished the Ministry of Health and Welfare and downgraded the primary healthcare department to a unit in the Ministry of Society. The changes caused strong opposition from Korean health and medical professions. The Korean Medical Society protested against the government's decision and waged a campaign to return the healthcare office to the ministry level. When the government restored the Ministry of Health in March 1949 under popular pressure, it did not restore the actual health administration to the level of American military government time. The South Korean government under Syngman Rhee prioritized military and economic affairs with dictatorial control. To make matters worse, when the U.S. military left, they took with them healthcare specialists and medical staff. As a result, more than half of the health personnel were lost in the Ministry of Health, the National Infectious Disease Research Institute, and the National Chemical Research Institute.[38]

The Korean War fundamentally changed the situation. The South Korean government revamped the health system by passing the National Health Care Law in September 1951 to handle the immediate urgent health needs of the war, particularly the control of infectious diseases and military medical relief. The law strengthened the medical license system, introduced a public physician system and improved the status of traditional medicine doctors. More importantly, it expanded health centers across the country to provide medical relief, administer infectious disease surveys and prevention, offer mother–child health work and health education and compile reports on vital statistics. The number of health centers increased to 406 by 1952, but many lacked trained staff and facilities, failing to provide basic health services.[39] In the meantime, the World Health Organization and the United Nations Korean Reconstruction Agency (UNKRA was an American agency despite the name) issued a report of detailed surveys of South Korean healthcare and health conditions. It recommended the establishment of a nationwide system of health clinic centers/units with an improved formula of operation to solve both short- and long-term needs.[40] The health mission of the WHO and the UNKRA was part of an overall collaboration between the South Korean government and the United States to achieve military victory of the Korean War, with economic modernization in agriculture and resource management, including introducing animal stocks of "pure breed, vaccinated, and free from major stock diseases."[41] Archival documents suggested the secrecy of the WHO–UNKRA's health mission during the Korean War. Scholars contended the possible link of the mission to the alleged use of germ warfare in China and North Korea by the United States during the Korean War.[42]

The new health clinic centers, which were modeled on the health centers created by the Rockefeller Foundation, were each supposed to have a doctor, a physician assistant, a public health nurse, several hygiene inspectors and a dozen of nurses and midwives in charge of all health matters, including disease prevention and medical treatment. In reality, the health clinics functioned poorly for lack of funding, facilities and trained personnel. Ordinary people, who fell ill while suffering war destruction and poverty, could not afford to see the doctors at the clinics or the use of expensive modern medicine. They had to rely on traditional medicine for health needs outside of the clinics. Traditional medicine, which was cheap and accessible, remained the main source of health and medical provisions for the majority of Koreans in times of poor economic situations.[43]

South Korea relied heavily on American and international economic aid and professional assistance after the Korean War. The massive American aid had an enormous impact on the economy and society of South Korea.[44] The International Cooperation Agency (which became USAID in 1961) alone sent South Korea more than a million dollars of aid each year in the 1950s, which was almost the same amount as the government budget for drugs, facilities and buildings.[45] In addition to the United States, the WHO significantly shaped South Korean government's health policies by involving in the rebuilding of health infrastructure in the 1950s and 1960s. When health clinics' facilities improved in the 1960s, people still shunned the service because of the arrogant attitude of the staff. According to the surveys conducted by the WHO and international aid agencies, more than half of the interviewed South Koreans mentioned that the arrogance of health staff was a major reason they did not go to the health clinics for help.[46] The military government under Park Chung-hee initiated laws for medical insurance for the purpose of increasing economic production in the 1960s, but it made little commitment of national resources to implementing the plan. Only after South Korea's economy took off in the 1970s–1980s did a national medical insurance system begin to be built with the passage of a series of health laws. South Korea followed the model of the Japanese health insurance system. In 1989, the National Health Service was launched, whereby all citizens would receive healthcare and medical treatment at medical centers with low costs, due to government subsidies.[47]

Park Yunjae's chapter investigates South Korea's development of public health with American aid in the Cold War and the influence of the Japanese model of medical insurance during the years of fast economic growth in the 1970s and 1980s. Against the background of international support, including those from the WHO and the UNICEF, Park examines the public-private partnership in anti-epidemic disease projects, especially the anti-tuberculosis work. His chapter demonstrates public enthusiasm and cooperation in expanding efforts of disease prevention and control, even when the South Korean government did not make a serious commitment to implementing healthcare plans with national resources. It also studies the changes in policies and laws that were related to the development of healthcare and public health. Drawing on the primary sources that he has researched over the years and his book, *Modern History of Medicine in Korea* (2021), Park Yunjae provides a comprehensive examination and interpretation of the connections between the support of international organizations and the development of healthcare and public health in South Korea.

Japan

Japan was occupied by the United States, similar to South Korea, in post-WWII. During the occupation from 1945 to 1952, the United States fundamentally shaped Japan's postwar recovery with drastic reforms in every aspect. The Supreme Commander for the Allied Powers initiated the creation of a new constitution along with land and industrial reforms to culturally and institutionally democratize and demilitarize Japan. The new constitution renounced the use of military force as national policy and held the government responsible to the people instead of to the emperor. The social and economic reforms defined by the SCAP emphasized equal rights for women, encouraged labor organizations and revived the economy with liberal progressive policies. However, when American politics shifted to the Cold War rivalry with the Soviet Union, the SCAP abandoned the ambitious plan of carrying out an America's Japan revolution and began to restrict labor activism and leftist groups. It relaxed the restrictions on war-time businesses and political leaders and let them return to power.[48]

The SCAP exercised the governing power by establishing a Japanese government in parallel to carry out the SCAP policies and programs. At the end of the war, Japan suffered food shortages, starvation and poverty. The situation was further exacerbated by widespread diseases, such as typhus, cholera, diphtheria, typhoid, tuberculosis, dysenteries and venereal disease. The SCAP was fully aware that public health work was of pivotal importance to the perceived success of the occupation.[49] It established a Public Health and Welfare Section (PHW) to handle the challenges of health and poverty, just like what the U.S. military government did in South Korea.

The health infrastructure in Japan, however, was very different from that in South Korea because Japan had built a national health insurance system for the mobilization of total war. When Japan started the war in China in the 1930s, it launched the movement to produce a physically fit population with the slogan "healthy soldiers, healthy people."[50] The aim was to build "a national defense state."[51] The Japanese government established the Health and Welfare Ministry, the National Health Insurance (NHI), and health centers in urban and rural areas. Japan also created the White-Collar Workers' Health Insurance, and the Seamen's Insurance during the war. The NHI programs were administered by private medical cooperatives and quasi-public National Health Insurance Associations in regions and municipalities. The Japanese government supervised the programs and provided financial support for the administrative costs. The expansion of health and medical services continued throughout the war years, with the construction of a health insurance system of near-universal coverage at the end of the war through those multiple programs.[52]

When the American occupation began in 1945, two thirds of the 10,000 healthcare associations were either bankrupt or inactive.[53] Despite the war destruction, Japan had an extensive health infrastructure that could be used by the occupation authorities. When the PHW administered national immunization programs, American military doctors often worked side by side with Japanese medical professionals.[54] The American occupation authorities relied on Japanese medical professionals and their cooperation in the implementation of postwar health policies and programs.

The head of the PHW was a hard-edged military doctor, Crawford F. Sams, who saw Japan as a primitive nation that needed reform.[55] This attitude about Japan was common among Americans during and after the war. Sams regarded Japan's health programs and services prior to the occupation "primitive in nature and ineffective in practice" and asserted that the American occupation was to give "modern concepts to Japan."[56] He claimed that the Japanese did not know what to do with the public health centers that were established by the RF in the 1930s. Sams sought the collaboration of the RF to work on Japan's health centers during the occupation. The RF, which had also built the Institute of Public Health in Japan in 1938, assumed a new postwar role in shaping up Japan's health programs by working with the SCAP.[57] When the Health Center Law was enacted in 1947, the aims appeared similar to that of the 1937 health center law, which ironically suggested continuity between the old and the new laws despite the war.[58]

The SCAP had the ambition to fundamentally reform Japan's healthcare system by integrating the various existing health insurance programs and centralizing the National Health Insurance into one unified comprehensive insurance system. Many civilian staff of the PHW had worked in the New Deal agencies of Franklin Roosevelt's administration, and they wanted to transform Japan in the progressive fashion of a New Deal.[59] They were also inspired by the postwar health reform in Britain, where a National Health Service was being built to create an integrated national health system. In April 1946, the "Advisory Commission on Labor First Interim Report" recommended that, given the existing separate programs for industrial wage earners, farmers, and self-employed in Japan, the PHW should consider "the feasibility of consolidating some or all of these programs into a unified, comprehensive social insurance system."[60] This progressive thrust to reform Japan was, however, fundamentally changed when American politics of the Cold War gained dominance and the SCAP took a conservative turn of reversing the course in Japan.

There was a drastic shift in political climate in Washington, D.C. two years after the end of WWII. The Truman administration had proposed a major postwar healthcare reform via the Wagner-Murray-Dingell bill in 1945, but Congress killed it with the strong lobby of the American Medical Association (AMA) and its allies. The opponents attacked Truman's healthcare reform as "socialized medicine" with government control. In the meantime, Cold War politics reshaped American domestic and foreign policies. When American domestic politics derailed Truman's health reform at home, the political powers directed their objections to the PHW's health reform in Japan as well. The AMA Mission to Japan in 1948 warned that government authority over medicine could lead to the return of a totalitarian government in Japan. They recommended that American occupation authorities promote a healthcare system that would closely resemble the one in the United States, that is, employment-based private insurance.[61] Sams of the PHW assured the AMA mission that no total nationalization of medicine would occur in Japan. The SCAP thereafter shifted policy priorities in the emerging Cold War and abandoned the plan to implement systematic health reform in Japan. The PHW eventually managed a few piecemeal changes in Japan's wartime fragmented health insurance system, leaving the financial burden of healthcare to be borne by the insured.[62] The PHW stated, in line with the new Cold War politics, that "compulsory national health insurance is not acceptable under SCAP policy."[63]

When the Japanese government was restored to power at the end of American occupation in 1952, it began to strengthen government authority over healthcare and tried to solidify the health insurance system toward universal healthcare, a process some Japanese scholars portrayed as a continuation from wartime, ignoring the postwar American episode.[64] The Japanese government reversed some of the PHW programs and policies that were not popular with the Japanese, namely, the termination of pensions for wounded Japanese soldiers, the rejection of segregated orphanages for mixed-race children, the suppression of medical reports on the effect of atomic bombs, the separation of the professions of medicine and pharmacy, and the nursing education reforms.[65] In 1956, the Japanese government passed the Health Insurance Amendment to initiate a new fee structure to address health equity and tighten the regulations of doctors who accepted health insurance payments. In 1958, the Japanese Parliament passed the National Health Insurance Amendment to make enrollment mandatory for people not covered by employment-based plans and to make municipalities cover all their residents. In 1961, Japan established universal health insurance to provide low-cost healthcare for all citizens. As Japan experienced the economic miracle of growth in the 1950s through the 1970s, the government increased spending on healthcare to reduce the costs of medical services and drugs. The various health insurance programs, however, retained the different benefits and premiums between the Health Insurance and the National Health Insurance. The merger of small towns and villages into bigger municipalities strengthened the financial resources, manpower and facilities of health at local level when national and local governments provided considerable funds and subsidies for healthcare.[66]

In his chapter, Takakazu Yamagishi investigates how the Cold War affected Japan's health insurance policies up to 1961 when universal healthcare was introduced. He pays special attention to the roles of medical associations and labor organizations in the negotiations of health programs within the existing institutional settings and political environment. His study illustrates how different institutional players as well as individuals contributed to the changes and continuity of health policies and health insurance programs, particularly when big businesses, the Japanese Medical Association and the Liberal Democratic Party formed a dominant power block to influence what was to change or not. The chapter explains the development of health insurance policies and programs before the end of WWII and analyzes the Cold War effect on health insurance politics and policies during the US-led occupation and the movement toward a universal health insurance system in Japan after the US occupation ended.

Between the Models: India and Indonesia

Between the socialist people's health and the capitalist private health insurance lay the health systems that combined public and private medical services in countries like India and Indonesia. After their independence from the British and the Dutch colonial rule, respectively, India and Indonesia guarded their sovereignty carefully to avoid ideological affiliations and alliances with either of the two superpowers in the Cold War rivalry. In fact, they led the Non-Aligned Movement at the 1955 Bandung Conference to carve out an independent third way to conduct international relations.[67] Their desire for neutrality and independence in international relations, however, was seriously eroded in the games of international aid and the contention of global power politics.

India

The national government of India established the Ministry of Health in 1947 after India gained independence from Britain. Like other Asian countries, India suffered major epidemic diseases, such as cholera, malaria, tuberculosis, smallpox, leprosy and plague, at the end of WWII.[68] The government of India made healthcare a priority in the five-year plan of national reconstruction, but the delivery of health programs was left to individual states of the federation. According to the constitution of India, the national government was responsible for ensuring the "right to health" for all people regardless of their socio-economic status, but each state was responsible for providing healthcare services for the people in the federal structure of the political system. In the construction of national health, the central government defined policies and provided a national strategic framework of programs and medical education. It was responsible for the administration of national disease control but delegated to individual states the duties of organizing and implementing disease prevention services. Consequently, huge discrepancies in disease control, quality and coverage of healthcare, and medical education emerged among the states and between urban centers and rural countryside.[69]

The threat of communicable diseases to national recovery prompted the national government to emphasize the importance of disease prevention and healthcare in national planning. India established a three-tiered system of primary healthcare as the foundation of national health for all people. At the lowest level were primary health centers to provide basic medical services, disease prevention, and health education. The next tier up was subdistrict centers to provide public health services. The top tier was hospitals to offer specialist services.[70] In the national five-year plans, health had a separate allocation, but it always received a low priority of funding. Studies of India's public health pointed out that the national government acknowledged people's right to health and the importance of public health service, but it rarely committed serious financial support to health construction and services. Instead, the government relied on international aid. The government also let the private provision of healthcare develop into a major force in the society. Widespread privatization led to the dominant role of the private sector in providing healthcare. Sunil Amrith argued that India's government never intended to eliminate the private provision of healthcare. In the 1950s through the 1970s, India witnessed under-investment and poor health infrastructure with low priority of government funding for public health. Even as India opted to be a liberal democratic state in its political orientation, public health was weak in the competition for national support and resources. Foreign aid became a significant source of health research and development. There was a huge gap between the expectations and the availability of health service in India.[71]

The government increasingly depended on international aid and external resources from both the United States and the Soviet Union. The United States contributed more than 50 percent of the costs of the malaria program between 1952 and 1958.[72] India also relied on the professional and financial assistance of the WHO and the RF.[73] The ruling elite in India emphasized scientific innovations and the techno approach in disease prevention. They targeted single diseases with techno-centric interventions but neglected general health services and health education of the people. Some studies indicated that few popular campaigns were carried out to raise people's awareness of health and disease prevention. The result was an "absence of any deep social awareness that health is a right and an entitlement of citizenship."[74] However, significant variations in fact existed in India, as individual states provided the actual organization of health programs and the implementation of health policies and services. For instance, Kerala state championed "people's right to health with political movement, which included political mobilization, local activism, public discussion of people's right to health via popular press of newspapers and magazines, and cooperative efforts, to achieve broad improvement of people's healthcare and services."[75]

India developed a mixed healthcare system with public and private healthcare providers. The public providers served only a small percentage of the population while the private providers overtook the majority. The shortage of health personnel and facilities and the lack of government commitment of financial resources to health development left the political commitment to health for all essentially an empty promise in those years. Domestic investments of national resources in health appeared less urgent when significant foreign aid was available in health and medical research. The private sector of medical and health services expanded significantly, but they were too expensive to be affordable for the majority of a large population.[76] The concept of democratic decentralization adopted by the Indian government shifted the responsibility for health to local people with little help from the central government. In the end, India's health system largely failed to provide health services to the people, except for the opening of some primary healthcare centers at the local level and some effect on the control of communicable diseases. Not until 1983 was the first National Health Policy of India formulated to emphasize the urgent need to establish a network of primary healthcare services. Extensive health service infrastructure was thereafter being developed with substantial numbers of healthcare personnel being trained.

To investigate the Cold War politics and preventive medicine in the early decades of independent India, Shirish N. Kavadi studies, in his chapter, the intertwined relations of foreign aid and virus research between 1950 and 1962. Situated in the larger context of the RF's global virus program and outreach, his chapter examines the RF's support of medical research, especially virus research in India, by founding the Virus Research Centre (VRC) in Poona (now Pune). His study details the objectives and scope of the virus research program in India and the use of research results in producing vaccines to tackle the outbreaks of epidemic diseases, such as the Kysanaur forest disease, during this time. The chapter analyzes the Indian government's responses to foreign aid and the controversies of virus research amidst the politicization of medical research and foreign aid. Kavadi makes a clear argument that the virus research in India was an essential aspect in the advancement of medical science. He emphasizes that the creation and sharing of medical knowledge are crucial to preventive medicine and public health in the world.

Indonesia

Patterns of central policy-making and local delivery of healthcare were seen in Indonesia as well during national reconstruction. After independence from the Dutch colonial rule in 1949, the new sovereign government of Indonesia made public health an important part of national reconstruction but delegated the delivery of health programs to local governments with limited financial and professional resources. Indonesia nationalized private hospitals and took control of health institutions and medical schools in establishing a national health system, but the government allowed physicians to keep their private practice on the side. Hans Pols points out that physicians became national doctors working in the state healthcare institutions after national independence. They strove for the right of people in obtaining physical and mental health and shaped Indonesia's healthcare approach by combining techno methods with social medicine. They emphasized medical technology and science in specialization and hospital-based care while promoting sanitation and public health measures.[77] Vivek Neelakantan argues that Indonesian health leaders believed that epidemic diseases were responsible for debilitating the capacity of the nation's workforce and resulting in lowered agricultural productivity and starvation. In their view, a strong and healthy population was vital in ensuring the prosperity of the nation.[78] Unlike the international agencies that correlated the prevalence of disease with poverty, Indonesian physicians saw diseases as caused by not poverty alone but rooted in socioeconomic conditions, political structures and the environment. The national health discourse after independence was to eradicate diseases to further the victories of the nation against poverty, illiteracy and poor health in the cultivation of a strong and healthy population.[79]

In fighting against disease and modernizing the nation, the Indonesian government sought international assistance as many other countries did. Both the United States and the Soviet Union expanded their international aid programs to gain influence in newly independent countries, and Indonesia worked with both of them. Moreover, international organizations such as the WHO, the United Nations Children's Emergency Fund and the South-East Asia Regional Office of the WHO significantly influenced Indonesia's health development.[80] In 1952, Indonesia's Ministry of Health adopted the suggestions made by the WHO's Expert Advisory Panel and presented a plan for the organization of healthcare for the country. The plan defined the delivery of healthcare at four local levels: hospital care in urban centers, auxiliary hospitals in districts, clinics in subdistricts and health posts in outer villages. Public health initiatives and education, and curative care were integrated at all four levels. Public health also became a compulsory component of medical curricula.[81] Indonesia launched campaigns against the four major epidemic diseases—tuberculosis, malaria, yaws and leprosy—that had plagued the people. Studies show that the anti-disease operation was ineffective and fragmented. Health leaders were unable to mobilize local people's participation in a truly public campaign to address the issues of socioeconomic conditions and change people's health knowledge, attitudes and behaviors.[82] The government mainly took the WHO's directive and centered on technical reliance on DDT and BCG, that is, the strategies of targeting specific diseases rather than a socioeconomic transformation in control of epidemic disease to solve health problems. The Health Ministry spent 90 percent of its budget on curative care and administration.[83] Large portions of the population remained malnourished and continued to suffer from epidemics such as smallpox, malaria, tuberculosis, trachoma, typhoid fever, leprosy and yaws. Several factors contributed to the ineffective health campaigns. Technically, Indonesia had limited health facilities and manpower with only a few health institutions and a small number of trained physicians. Economically, Indonesia faced daunting challenges to rebuild the infrastructure that was destroyed by the war and to get the economy back to normal growth. Politically, since independence, the country "experienced continuous political instability, internal conflict, and external pressure to such an extent that government rarely held power more than a year."[84]

Indonesia, however, did not blindly follow the instruction of international aid agencies, even as it welcomed assistance from any country and any international organization. As a leader of the Non-Aligned Movement, Indonesia guarded its sovereignty with national policies of self-sufficiency and not being dependent on any one country for assistance. It resisted the American pressures on free market and trade, abolition of tariffs and free reign for American companies. In the late 1950s, Soekarno gradually turned away from the American model and shifted toward the models of the Soviet Union and China.[85] Such a change led to tensions with the United States and the coup of 1965, which ended Soekarno's rule.

After 1967, the Soeharto government put emphasis on developing a free-market economy with the American model, but the government played a significant role in sponsoring enterprises. This policy and strategy of national development widened social and economic inequalities, as the growth of national economy increased. In the 1970s, the government began the construction of primary health centers (*puskesmas*) in every subdistrict or area with a population of 30,000 to 50,000.[86] Consequently, Indonesia developed a healthcare system of public and private providers. The public system was administered at different levels, with the central, provincial and district governments taking on different responsibilities. The central Ministry of Health was responsible for the management of some tertiary and specialist hospitals, provisions for strategic direction, setting up standards and regulations and ensuring the availability of financial and human resources. Provincial governments were responsible for the management of provincial-level hospitals, providing technical oversight, monitoring district health services and coordinating cross-district health issues within the province. District/municipal governments were responsible for the management of district/city hospitals and the district public health network of community health centers and associated sub-district facilities.[87]

Vivek Neelakantan's chapter examines the health policies of Indonesia throughout the Cold War era and analyzes the changing interpretation of public health in national reconstruction from the Soekarno era (Old Order, 1949–1966) to the Soeharto government (New Order, 1966–1998). It pays special attention to Indonesia's policies toward international aid and its efforts to maintain an independent foreign policy under Soekarno before the shift to adopt the American model of economic development during Soeharto's government. Neelakantan explains that during the Soekarno era the health of the people played an important role in the completion of national revolution and the establishment of a socialist society. During the Soeharto era, public health was not perceived as a security risk for the state. The central government under Soeharto implemented health policies such as family planning down to the village level, and charged significant user fees at health centers in local communities. Neelakantan argues that the overarching theme of health policy across the Old and New Orders was national development (*pembangunan*), but the paths to which were interpreted very differently by the Old and

New Orders. The chapter makes an explicit connection to current public health concerns by investigating how epidemic diseases such as H5N1 influenza and COVID-19 were handled by the decentralized health administration of Indonesia.

Conclusion

The development of public health and healthcare systems in the six Asian countries during the Cold War demonstrated the interactions and negotiations between domestic policy interests and international aid influence. Although the United States and the Soviet Union promoted competing models of modernization and national development, the political system and national priorities of each individual country shaped the paths to national health construction with ideological justification and pragmatic consideration. The chapters in this book provide an illuminating comparative study of the different paths of national development and health construction that were intertwined with Cold War international politics and domestic socioeconomic transformations.

Public health not only achieved the control of diseases and improvement of people's health but also served the political and social goals of promoting particular national visions and ideologies for development in each country. In socialist China and North Korea, the state planned, organized and funded national healthcare as an integral part of the socioeconomic transformation of the society, promoting universal free healthcare for the people and social equality. In capitalist Japan and South Korea, healthcare was left to the operation of private enterprises as businesses, with the promotion of freedom and individual choices. The commitment of the state to people's health in China and North Korea contrasted with the market approach to public health in Japan and South Korea. However, the state in Japan and in South Korea, motivated by the desire to boost economic growth and political popularity, increasingly intervened with laws and policies to promote and regulate health programs. The government in Japan and South Korea provided substantial subsidies to healthcare to address the problems of affordability and accessibility, especially when their economic growth reached a certain level. In the case of Japan, the government committed significant funding for national healthcare to achieve the goal of universal healthcare since the 1960s. In South Korea, the government increased subsidies to national health programs since the 1980s to lower the costs for individuals.

The Non-Aligned countries of India and Indonesia tried to realize their national visions of health as the right of the people but encountered constant alterations of international aid and influence, in addition to domestic inability to deliver healthcare for the people in the early decades after independence. By staying neutral to the Cold War rivalry of the two superpowers, India and Indonesia welcomed aid and assistance from all sides. India relied significantly on international aid in medical research and disease control during the Cold

War, which contributed to the lack of commitment of the national government to allocating national resources to health programs. Indonesia welcomed international aid and resisted external pressures on its independent policies of national development during the Soekarno era (1949–1966). That policy changed when Indonesia had a coup and Soekarno was edged out of power. With the establishment of the New Order, the Soeharto government in Indonesia followed the American model of economic development but with significant state intervention. People had to pay significant user fees to get health services.

National interests and local health and economic conditions proved especially relevant to the development of national health in each country, even though international influence and aid complicated the process of national reconstruction during the Cold War. With the influence of different political ideologies and competing models of modernization, Asian countries took different paths to health construction with particular national visions of political aspirations, economic prosperity, and social transformation. National health developed in line with the political and social goals of the national projection by the state. Despite the superpowers' rivalry in the world and their influence on national health development of Asian countries, local conditions of health infrastructure and practices as well as health knowledge proved crucial to the delivery of health programs in each country. The chapters analyze the tensions between domestic policies and foreign aid. More importantly, they demonstrate the creative adaptation of the countries to domestic needs and the changing international politics to advance national health visions. Kavadi's chapter on India's virus research shows there was health collaboration in medical research and disease prevention across the Cold War camps, despite their ideological differences. It is most relevant today, as Kavadi points out, that global health requires international cooperation and collaboration for the benefit of humankind.

Notes

1 Odd Arned Westad, *The Global Cold War: Third World Interventions and the Making of Our Times* (Cambridge: Cambridge University Press, 2011).
2 On modernization theory, see Michael Latham, *Modernization as Ideology: American Social Science and "Nation Building" in the Kennedy Era* (Chapel Hill: University of North Carolina Press, 2003); Nils Gilman, *Mandarins of the Future: Modernization Theory in Cold War America* (Baltimore: The Johns Hopkins University Press, 2007); David C. Engerman, Nils Gilman, Mark H. Haefele and Michael E. Latham, eds., *Staging Growth: Modernization, Development and the Global Cold War* (Amherst: University of Massachusetts Press, 2003); and Bradley Simpson, *Economists with Guns: Authoritarian Development and U.S.-Indonesian Relations* (California: Stanford University Press, 2010).
3 János Kornai, *The Socialist System: The Political Economy of Communism* (Oxford: Blackwell, 1992); Corinna R. Unger, *International Development: A Postwar History* (Bloomsbury Academic, 2018); and Thomas P. Bernstein, "The Socialist Modernization of China Between Soviet Model and National Specificity

1949–1960s" in *The Cambridge History of Communism*, eds. Norman Naimark, Silvio Pons and Sophie Quinn-Judge (Cambridge: Cambridge University Press, 2017).

4 John Lewis Gaddis, *The United States and the Origins of the Cold War, 1941–1947* (New York: Columbia University Press, 2000); and Michael Schaller, *American Occupation of Japan: The Origins of the Cold War in Asia* (Oxford: Oxford University Press, 1987).

5 Richard Bernstein, *China 1945: Mao's Revolution and America's Fateful Choice* (New York: Vintage, 2015); and Daniel Kurtz-Phelan, *The China Mission: George Marshall's Unfinished War, 1945–1947* (New York: W. W. Norton & Company, 2018).

6 Natasa Miskovic, Harald Fischer-Tiné, Nada Boskovska, eds., *The Non-Aligned Movement and the Cold War Delhi – Bandung – Belgrade* (London: Routledge, 2014).

7 David C. Engerman, *The Price of Aid: The Economic Cold War in India* (Boston: Harvard University Press, 2018); Vivek Neelakantan, *Science, Public Health and Nation-Building in Soekarno-Era Indonesia* (Newcastle upon Tyne: Cambridge Scholars Publishing, 2017); Bradley Simpson, *Economists with Guns*; and Bipan Chandra, *India Since Independence* (Penguin Random House India, 2008).

8 President Truman spoke of four courses of action in international relations by the United States: (1) support of the United Nations, (2) programs for world economic recovery, (3) the strengthening of freedom-loving nations against the dangers of communist aggression, and (4) sharing the benefits of American scientific advances (the Point Four program). ("Inaugural Address of the President," *The U.S. Department of State Bulletin* 20, January 30, 1949), 125.

9 Liping Bu, *MAKING THE WORLD LIKE US: Education, Cultural Expansion, and the American Century* (CT: Praeger, 2003); Walter L. Hixson, *Parting the Curtain: Propaganda, Culture, and the Cold War, 1945-1961* (New York: St. Martin's Press, 1997); Jessica Trisko Darden, *Aiding and Abetting: U.S. Foreign Assistance and State Violence* (CA: Stanford University Press, 2019).

10 Marcos Cueto, "International Health, the Early Cold War and Latin America," *CBMH/BCHM (Canadian Bulletin of Medical History)* 25, no. 1 (2008): 17–41.

11 Daniel Kurtz-Phelan, *The China Mission*.

12 Robert P. Newman, *Owen Lattimore and the "Loss" of China* (CA: University of California Press, 1992); Tang Tsou, *America's Failure in China, 1941–50* (Chicago: University of Chicago Press, 1963); Richard Bernstein, *China 1945*; Kevin Peraino, *A Force So Swift: Mao, Truman, and the Birth of Modern China, 1949* (New York: Crown, 2018).

13 Mary Augusta Brazelton, *Mass Vaccination: Citizens' Bodies and State Power in Modern China* (Cornell: Cornell University Press, 2019).

14 Liping Bu, *Public Health and the Modernization of China, 1865–2015* (London: Routledge, 2017).

15 Liping Bu, "Anti-Malaria Campaigns and Socialist Reconstruction of China, 1950–1980," *East Asian History* 39 (2014): 117–130.

16 David Hipgrave, "Communicable Disease Control in China: From Mao to Now," *Journal of Global Health* 1.2 (December 2011): 224–238.

17 Lorenz M. Lüthi, *The Sino-Soviet Split: Cold War in the Communist World* (Princeton, NJ: Princeton University Press, 2008).

18 *Collections of Documents on Rural Health Work, 1951–2000* (Ministry of Health, PRC, 2001).

19 Shin Dong-won, "Public Health and People's Health: Contrasting the Paths of Healthcare Systems in South and North Korea, 1945–60," in *Public Health and*

National Reconstruction in Post-War Asia: International Influences, Local Transformations, eds. Liping Bu and Ka-che Yip (London: Routledge, 2015), 91–94.

20 Hong Sun-won, *History of Public Health in North Korea* (Pyengyang: Kwahak PaekgwaSajŏn Ch'ulpansa, 1981), 415, cited in Shin Dong-won, "Public Health and People's Health." 95–96.

21 Jin-hyouk Kim and Mi-ra Moon, "The Socialist Camp's North Korean Medical Support and Exchange (1945–1958): Between Learning from the Soviet Union and Independent Course," *Korean Journal of Medical History* 28, no. 1 (2019): 139–190.

22 Shin Dong-won, "Public Health and People's Health," 97.

23 Shin Dong-won, "How Four Different Political Systems Have Shaped the Modernization of Traditional Korean Medicine between 1900 and 1960," *Historia Scientiarum* 7, no. 3 (2008): 238.

24 Jin-hyouk Kim and Mi-ra Moon, "The Socialist Camp's North Korean Medical Support."

25 This was the period when China's relations with the Soviet Union deteriorated and China suffered significant economic setbacks in the wake of the Great Leap Forward and the Soviet withdrawal of aid.

26 John Grundy, "History, International Relations, and Public Health—The Case of the Democratic People's Republic of Korea 1953–2015," *Korea's Economy* 31, Part IV: Sectoral Conditions in North Korea (Washington, D.C.: Korea Economic Institute, 2017): 53.

27 Eom Ju-Hyun, *History of the Formation of North Korean Healthcare System, 1945–1970* (Sunin, 2021).

28 Sunyoung Pak, Daniel Schwekendiek, and Hee Kayoing Kim, "Height and Living Standards in North Korea, 1930s–1980s," *Economic History Review*, 64, S1 (2011): 142–158.

29 Jin-hyouk Kim and Mi-ra Moon, "The Socialist Camp's North Korean Medical Support."

30 John Grundy, "History, International Relations, and Public Health."

31 Liping Bu, Darwin H. Stapleton and Ka-che Yip, eds., *Science, Public Health and the State in Modern Asia* (London: Routledge, 2012); John Farley, *To Cast out Disease. A History of the International Health Division of the Rockefeller Foundation, 1913–1951*(New York: Oxford University Press, 2004).

32 John DiMoia, *Reconstructing Bodies: Biomedicine, Health, and Nation-Building in South Korea Since 1945* (Stanford, CA: Stanford University Press, 2013).

33 Kornel Chang, "Independence without Liberation: Democratization as Decolonization Management in U.S.-Occupied Korea, 1945–1948," *Journal of American History* 107, no. 1 (June 2020): 77–106.

34 Shin Jwa-seŏp, "The Policy of the United States Army Military Government in Korea toward Public Health and Medicine in Occupied South Korea," *Korean Journal of Medical History* 9, no. 2 (2000): 212–232; Crawford F. Sams and Zabelle Zakarian, *Medic: The Mission of an American Military Doctor in Occupied Japan and Wartorn Korea* (London: Routledge, 1997).

35 Choe Chai-chang, *American Medicine in Korean Medical History* (Seoul: Yonglim Cardinal, 1996), cited in Shin Dong-won, "Public Health and People's Health," 102.

36 Jŏng Sŏn-tae and Kim Hyen-sik eds., *Voices Appeared in Political Pamphlets Just after Liberation* (Seoul: Somyengch'ulpan, 2011), cited in Shin Dong-wen, "Public Health and People's Health," 103.

37 Shin Jwa-seŏp, "The Policy of the United States Army Military Government in Korea," 223.

38 Shin Dong-won, "Public Health and People's Health," 103–104.
39 Ibid., 104.
40 Kyuri Kim and Buhm Soon Park, "Infrastructure-Building for Public Health: The World Health Organization and Tuberculosis Control in South Korea, 1945–1963," *Korean Journal of Medical History* 28, no. 1 (2019): 89–138.
41 Lisa M. Brady, "Sowing War, Reaping Peace: United Nations Resource Development Programs in the Republic of Korea, 1950–1953," *Journal of Asian Studies* 77, no. 2 (May 2018): 351–363.
42 Jane Sung Ha Kim, "Leprosy in Korea: A Global History," PhD dissertation (University of California, Los Angeles, 2012), chapter 5.
43 Shin Dong-won, "How Four Different Political Systems Have Shaped the Modernization of Traditional Korean Medicine between 1900 and 1960," 225–241.
44 Gregg Brazinsky, *Nation Building in South Korea: Koreans, Americans and the Making of a Democracy* (Chapel Hill: University of North Carolina Press 2009).
45 Shin Dong-won, "Public Health and People's Health," 106.
46 Kyuri Kim, "The Triad that Brought Madras to South Korea: Infrastructure-Building for Tuberculosis Control in Post-Colonial South Korea." Paper presented at the 15th International Conference on the History of Science in East Asia, Chonbuk National University, Jeonju, Republic of Korea, August 19–23, 2019.
47 Shin Dong-won, *History of Modern Medicine and Public Health in Korea* (Hanul, 1997); and John DiMoia, *Reconstructing Bodies.*
48 Theodore Cohen, *Remaking Japan: The American Occupation as New Deal* (London: Collier Macmillan, 1987).
49 Christopher Aldous and Akihito Suzuki, *Reforming Public Health in Occupied Japan, 1945–1952: Alien Prescriptions?* (London: Routledge, 2012), 8.
50 G. J. Kasza, "War and Welfare Policy in Japan," *Journal of Asian Studies* 61, no. 2 (2002): 417–435.
51 Ibid.
52 G. J. Kasza, "War and Welfare Policy in Japan;" Yoneyuki Sugita, "Universal Health Insurance: The Unfinished Reform of Japan's Healthcare System," in *Democracy in Occupied Japan: The U.S. Occupation and Japanese Politics and Society*, eds. Mark E. Caprio and Yoneyuki Sugita (London: Routledge, 2007).
53 Takakazu Yamagishi, *War and Health Insurance Policy in Japan and the United States: World War II to Postwar Reconstruction* (Baltimore: The Johns Hopkins University Press, 2011), 115.
54 Sey Nishimura, "Promoting Health during the American Occupation of Japan: The Public Health Section, Kyoto Military Government Team, 1945–1949," *American Journal of Public Health* 98, no. 3 (March 2008), 424–434.
55 Crawford F. Sams, "American Public Health Administration Meets the Problems of the Orient in Japan," *American Journal of Public Health and the Nation's Health* 42, no. 5 (1952): 557–65; Cawford F. Sams and Zabelle Zakarian, *Medic.*
56 Sams, "Japan's New Public Health Program," *Military Government Journal* 1, no. 11 (Sept–Oct 1948), 9–14.
57 Kazumi Noguchi, "Impact of Government-Foundation Cooperation: Health Care System Development in Post-War Japan," in *Public Health and National Reconstruction in Post-War Asia*, 112–131; Aiko Takeuchi-Demirci, 'From Race Biology to Population Control: The Rockefeller Foundation's "Public Health" Projects in Japan, 1920s–1950s,' in *Science, Public Health and the State in Modern Asia*, 113–128.
58 Christopher Aldous and Akihito Suzuki, *Reforming Public Health in Occupied Japan*, 171.
59 Theodore Cohen, *Remaking Japan.*
60 Takakazu Yamagishi, *War and Health Insurance Policy in Japan and the United States*, 119.

61 American Medical Association, "Report of the Mission of the American Medical Association," 1948.
62 Takakazu Yamagishi, *War and Health Insurance Policy in Japan and the United States*, 118–128.
63 Sugita, "Universal Health Insurance," 163.
64 Naoki Ikegami, Byung-Kwang Yoo, Hideki Hashimoto, Masatoshi Matsumoto et al, "Japanese Universal Health Coverage: Evolution, Achievements, and Challenges," *The Lancet* 378, no. 9796 (September 2011): 1106–1115; Takakazu Yamagishi, "Health Insurance Politics of Japan in the 1940s and the 1950s: The Japan Medical Association and Policy Development," *Journal of International and Advanced Japanese Studies* 9 (March 2017): 193–204.
65 Sey Nishimura, "Promoting Health in American-Occupied Japan: Resistance to Allied Public Health Measures, 1945–1952," *American Journal of Public Health* 99, no. 8 (August 2009): 1364–1375.
66 Yasuki Kobayashi, "Five Decades of Universal Health Insurance Coverage in Japan: Lessons and Future Challenges," *Japanese Medical Association Journal* 52, no. 4 (July/August 2009): 263–268.
67 Natasa Miskovic, Harald Fischer-Tiné and Nada Boskovska, eds., *The Non-Aligned Movement and the Cold War*.
68 D. M. Gupte, V. Ramachandran and R. K. Mutatkar, "Epidemiological Profile of India: Historical and Contemporary Perspectives," *Journal of Biosciences* 26, no. 4 (November 2001): 437–464.
69 Sanjoy Bhattacharya, *Expunging Variola: The Control and Eradication of Smallpox in India, 1947-1977* (Hyderabad: Orient Longman, 2006); and Vivek Neelakantan, "Tuberculosis Control in Postcolonial South India and Southeast Asia: Fractured Sovereignties in International Health, 1948–1960," *Wellcome Open Research* 2, no. 4 (2018): 1–18, https://doi.org/10.12688/wellcomeopenres.10544.2.
70 The ideas of a three-tiered primary healthcare system came from the 1946 Bhore Committee Report and the 1948 Sokhey Committee Report that recommended significant reforms of the national health system of India to provide a comprehensive healthcare of preventive and curative medicine for all people. See Shirish N. Kavadi, "Medicine, Philanthropy, and Nationhood: Tensions of Different Visions in India," in *Public Health and National Reconstruction in Post-War Asia*, 132–153.
71 Sunil S. Amrith, *Decolonizing International Health: South and Southeast Asia, 1930–1965* (Basingstoke: Palgrave Macmillan, 2006) and "Health in India since Independence," BWPI Working Paper 79 (Brooks World Poverty Institute, University of Manchester, 2009), 1–26.
72 Sunil S. Amrith, "Health in India since Independence," 13.
73 Vivek Neelakantan, ed., *The Geopolitics of Health in South and Southeast Asia: Perspectives from the Cold War to COVID-19* (London: Routledge, 2023).
74 Sunil S. Amrith, "Health in India since Independence," 14.
75 Ibid., 17–19.
76 Imrana Qadeer, "Health Care Systems in Transition III: India, Part I. The Indian Experience," *Journal of Public Health Medicine* 22, no. 1 (March 2000): 25–32.
77 Hans Pols, *Nurturing Indonesia: Medicine and Decolonisation in the Dutch East Indies* (Cambridge: Cambridge University Press, 2018), 204–207.
78 Vivek Neelakantan, *Science, Public Health and Nation-Building in Soekarno-Era Indonesia*.
79 Vivek Neelakantan, "The Campaign against the Big Four Endemic Diseases and Indonesia's Engagement with the WHO during the Cold War 1950s," in *Public Health and National Reconstruction in Post-War Asia*, 154–174.

80 Vivek Neelakantan, *Science, Public Health and Nation-Building in Soekarno-Era Indonesia.*

81 Hans Pols, *Nurturing Indonesia,* 209–213.

82 Vivek Neelakantan, "The Campaign against the Big Four," 154–174.

83 Hans Pols, *Nurturing Indonesia,* 211.

84 Ibid., 206.

85 Ibid., 209.

86 Yodi Mahendradhata et al., "The Republic of Indonesia Health System Review," *Health Systems in Transition* 7, no. 1 (World Health Organization, Regional Office for South-East Asia, 2017), 22–23.

87 Ibid., xxv–xxvi.

1 "Taking Our Own Road"

Building the People's Health in Socialist China

Liping Bu

Introduction

"The national liberation war has been won, but national wounds have not yet been healed. Scientific knowledge of health has not yet been popularized. Natural disasters and famine have resulted in the spread of epidemic diseases."[1] Such was the urgent situation of disease control and national health reconstruction when the People's Republic of China (PRC) was founded in 1949. People's health was an important part of national recovery and reconstruction. The new state aspired to build a new China with social justice and equality. The improvement of people's health and well-being constituted a foundation of the overall transformation of the society from the old to the new. Moreover, public health was essential to the delivery of a better society that the Communist-led revolution had been advocating. The road to national recovery and reconstruction, however, was filled with the challenges of widespread poverty, rampant epidemic diseases, broken infrastructures and a collapsed financial and economic system in the wake of decades of destructive wars.

The founding of the People's Republic of China coincided with the increasing rivalry between the two superpowers, as the United States and the Soviet Union engaged in a Cold War to reshape the world order. The superpowers promoted competing models of national development and modernization that were underlined with contrasting ideologies. The bipolar divergence divided the world into two camps—one with the United States leading the capitalist camp and the other with the Soviet Union leading the communist camp. The Cold War affected many countries, especially the direction of development of new sovereign nations. When the Chinese Communists defeated the Nationalists in the civil war and established the People's Republic of China, the United States was "alarmed" over China's fall to communism. The Republicans blamed the Democrats for "the loss of China" in typical American politics of finger-pointing. In the meantime, the United States continued the support for Chiang Kai-Shek's Nationalist regime in Taiwan with economic and military aid while obstructing Mao Zedong's Communist government on the mainland with economic sanctions and diplomatic non-recognition. The American isolation policies only helped push the PRC

DOI: 10.4324/9781003318163-2

toward the Soviet Union for support. The Soviet Union provided China with economic aid and technical support, while China followed the Soviet model to build a socialist society. China strengthened relations with the Soviet Union in the face of the U.S. sanctions and hostilities by signing the Sino-Soviet Treaty of Friendship, Alliance and Mutual Assistance in 1950.

The United States and China went on to have a military confrontation in the Korean War, where they fought against each other on the battlefields in support of the opposing sides in the conflict. The direct military clash in Korea meant no return for normal China–U.S. relations. In contrast, the Sino-Soviet relationship blossomed. With economic aid and technical support to China, the Soviet Union influenced Chinese industry, education, health, and cultural life in the 1950s. Over 11,000 Soviet scientists and technicians worked in China, and about 1,000 of them worked in the fields of education and health.[2] Russian replaced English as the first foreign language to learn in China. Chinese health and medical science, in this larger context, made an epistemological shift from the Anglo-American tradition to the Soviet model. Chinese intellectuals, medical doctors and scientists began to learn from the Soviet Union and reform their old ideas and values.[3] Chinese medical schools, following the Soviet model, redesigned the curricula to shorten the years of training for health professionals. The Soviet medical system "has three broad categories of health personnel: highly specialized physicians with extensive training; feldshers [similar to assistant physicians], who now have 3 to 4 years of medical education; and public health technicians."[4] In preventive medicine, China adopted a holistic, multipronged social approach to tackle major epidemic diseases at once instead of the techno method of targeting individual diseases that was popular in the United States and promoted by the World Health Organization (WHO). Chinese health services emphasized the five main areas that affected public health, that is, labor hygiene, food hygiene, environmental hygiene, school hygiene, and radiation hygiene.[5] Learning from the Soviet Union but drawing on Chinese experiences, China established the Health and Epidemic Prevention Stations as centers to fight diseases at local levels. More schools of public health were established at medical universities to train public health professionals. The enthusiasm to learn from the Soviet Union was short-lived, however, when Sino-Soviet relations deteriorated in the late 1950s and fell into open hostility in the 1960s. China's tensions with the United States, in the meantime, did not diminish. In fact, China faced simultaneously both sanctions and isolation by the United States and the withdrawal of economic and technical assistance by the Soviet Union. In this context of the Cold War with both superpowers, China took an independent and self-reliant road of socialist nation-building. It should be noted that even with prominent Soviet influence in the 1950s, China had demonstrated a characteristically Chinese model of national development and health reconstruction that was informed by Chinese circumstances and shaped by the guiding principles of national health policies.

Chinese leaders laid out the construction of the people's health with a strong determination of self-reliance when access to international assistance and technology was limited. National health work concentrated on the areas of fighting major epidemic diseases, protecting women's and children's health, improving ethnic minority people's health facilities and services, and protecting industrial workers' health. The government made special efforts to build medical and health services in rural and remote regions that had previously no access to modern medicine. The new health programs aimed at not only improving individuals' health but also strengthening the foundation of national economic development and winning popular support for the new state. In addition to the importance of people's well-being, the social and economic benefits of people's health were significant, as the improvement of people's health would ensure the undertakings of economic recovery and national defense as well as people's trust in the government.

Delivering the people's health and building a socialist society went hand in hand with China's national reconstruction during the Cold War. Health work was integrated into the general planning of social and economic recovery and development. The people's health, therefore, was a long-term commitment of the state to the well-being of the people. From the perspective of economic development, good health of the people was essential to economic productivity and national reconstruction of a prosperous China. Government officials and health professionals aspired to achieve better health for all the people, even though the country faced severe shortages of health personnel and facilities as well as financial and technical difficulties.

Public discourse and the media hailed the people's health as a demonstration of the superiority of the socialist system over the capitalist system. The main principles of national health policies defined the people's health as serving the workers, peasants and soldiers and making prevention the top priority. Large numbers of medical and health workers were trained in various types of programs at different technical levels. The government established many hospitals, created health institutes for women and children, and constructed nationwide networks of health and disease prevention. People were mobilized to participate in health campaigns as active agents to fight disease. In addition to extensive scale of vaccination, the health movement promoted personal and industrial hygiene, environmental sanitation, clean water sources, waste management, agricultural irrigation and reengineering of the ecosystems.

This chapter aims to enhance the understanding of the fundamental transformation of China in the Cold War during the 1950s through the 1970s via an examination of the various efforts to construct the people's health and build a socialist society. The study analyzes the influence of the Soviet Union and the tensions of the Cold War in affecting health policies and programs in China, along with political and social movements. It delineates the diverse programs of urban and rural healthcare and explores the political and social meanings of people's health. The training of barefoot doctors and the formation of rural medical cooperatives constituted the most significant development of health infrastructure in China. This chapter shows that even with the Soviet influence in the 1950s, China had carved out an independent road of socialist development that emphasized the building of rural and basic-level infrastructure and health services for the people during the different stages of socialist development.

Defining the People's Health: Policies and Programs

The people's health was defined by the principles of national health policies at the First National Health Conference in August 1950 as serving the needs of workers, peasants and soldiers and emphasizing disease prevention as the priority. A third principle of uniting Chinese and Western medicine was added after Chairman Mao Zedong wrote to the Conference with the call "to unite all the health and pharmaceutical personnel of old and new as well as Western and Chinese medicine, to form a solid united front and work hard for the development of the great people's health."[6] Those three principles reflected the national health aspirations, with the continuity of pre-1949 health practices conducted by the Communist-governed regions in serving the people and relying on traditional Chinese medicine.[7] A fourth principle of mass health movement was formed during the Korean War time.

In addition to the principles of national health policies, the First Health Conference also specified four major areas of immediate tasks: (1) strengthening and expanding basic health units; (2) readjusting public and private relationships in regard to medical, pharmaceutical and health institutions; (3) uniting medical and pharmaceutical groups for mutual aid and study; and (4) expanding health education and training of health workers at all levels.[8] The health principles and tasks provided the guidance and framework for the early programs of national health reconstruction.

Epidemic diseases were rampant in many parts of China when the PRC was established. More than twenty major epidemics were plaguing the Chinese people, such as smallpox, plague, cholera, typhus, typhoid fever, tuberculosis, tetanus, hookworm, schistosomiasis, kala-azar, meningitis, malaria, measles, polio, diphtheria, polio, leprosy, filariasis, and venereal disease. The diseases deprived cities and villages of productive population, causing extensive human suffering, and hundreds of thousands of deaths. Moreover, poverty, unsanitary conditions, malnutrition, and unhealthy habits further contributed to the spread of diseases and loss of lives. Protecting the health of 600 million Chinese people was a daunting task in 1950 when the country was suffering severe shortages of financial resources and lacked health manpower and facilities.

In order to address the multifaceted challenges, the government concentrated on fighting major epidemic diseases all at once in a coordinated manner across administrative departments, and integrated health programs into the national economic and social development plans to tackle the socioeconomic causes of diseases. Various government ministries, such as health, education, propaganda, industries, and agriculture, coordinated to mobilize the people to take part in health campaigns. Professional and social organizations, such as the Red Cross, the National Federation of Women, and the Labor Union, joined the movement to mobilize people of all walks of life and school children to kill pests and reduce diseases. The central government sent disease-prevention teams to work with local health workers. They would converge on epidemic-affected areas, combining the preventive methods of hygiene and sanitation with vaccination and treatment. As many places did not have basic health facilities, the prevention teams would set up mobile vaccination stations on the street to vaccinate people. They also built delousing stations with showers for people to use to improve personal hygiene and tackle typhus and relapsing fever.

Sanitation and hygiene were carried out in the general socioeconomic programs such as city planning and urban reconstruction, land reclamation, and transformation of ecosystems. People were mobilized to fill up dirty ponds and ditches and dredge rivers to reduce diseases such as malaria, kala-azar, and schistosomiasis. Cities and towns cleaned up the wartime debris and trash in mass campaigns. Opium addicts and prostitutes were rehabilitated to become healthy and productive citizens. Big cities conducted campaigns to clean up slums and shantytowns that were the eyesore of old China, as in the case of Longxugou of Beijing and Zhaojiabang of Shanghai. New neighborhoods were built, instead, with new water and sewage systems, and streets and residential buildings were lined with green trees.[9] The change of shantytowns symbolized the fundamental transformation of the old broken China into a new healthy China with great prospects.[10]

Health workers used all means available, such as hygiene, vaccination and treatment, to combat disease and improve people's health. They conducted health campaigns, educated people about disease and health, and illustrated the methods of disease prevention. Mass vaccination was carried out on an extensive scale against communicable diseases such as smallpox, cholera, and plague, the three most devastating diseases widespread in China.[11] About half of the total population of 600 million were vaccinated against smallpox in the first two years of the PRC. As a result, incidence of smallpox in 1951 was 90 percent less than in 1950.[12] By 1952, more than 512 million people had received vaccination against smallpox.[13] By 1963, China achieved the extraordinary success of total eradication of smallpox, a feat that was twenty years ahead of the world, without the assistance of WHO during the Cold War. In the prevention of cholera, Chinese health workers provided inoculations for people in the regions of contagion. More importantly, they made great efforts to mobilize people to clean up garbage and improve sanitation to ensure clean water sources. The government strengthened quarantine services along the communication and transportation lines as well. Sanitation campaigns together with vaccinations effectively brought the cholera epidemic under control.[14] In the prevention of plague, health workers encouraged people to catch rats and kill fleas in addition to taking anti-plague vaccination. The health campaigns, which were coordinated by various government departments, proved effective in controlling plague and even eradicating bubonic plague in certain regions. By the mid-1950s, bubonic plague was no longer a menace to the lives of Chinese people. China's experiences in the control and prevention of widespread epidemics indicated that it was important to have coordinated collaborations across sectors with community participation in order to achieve effective results of disease control. They demonstrated that disease prevention must not be separated from the overall socioeconomic improvement of people's life.

Existing health professions and institutions were consolidated and expanded, as many more new health workers were trained by using the Soviet model. Large numbers of health workers were trained to provide basic health services, particularly in rural areas. In 1951, the Health Ministry issued the "Specific Measures to Implement the Work of Rural Basic Health Organizations" to expand basic health personnel. The document defined basic health personnel as health workers, midwives (and assistants), and assistant nurses. Candidates were recruited from "sons and daughters of peasants and workers, elementary school teachers including rural elementary school teachers and private school students without gender discrimination."[15] "Midwives and assistant nurses should be recruited from old-style midwives, female elementary school graduates, female factory workers, rural women and elementary school teachers."[16] After they were selected, the recruits would undergo a short training program without leaving their current job. Health workers were expected to be devoted to serving the people. Village health workers were trained at town and district health stations or at the county hospitals. They focused on learning preventive medicine, first aid, and women's and children's health. Mothers' health and the control of newborn and puerperal infections were given special attention. The Health Ministry provided the curriculum, which defined half a year for the training of midwives and assistant nurses and eight weeks for the training of other health personnel. In the meantime, about 750,000 old-style midwives were retrained, and more than 2,380 women's and children's health centers were established by 1952. "No other type of medical facility increased at this rate, and a major result was the decline in neonatal tetanus, down from 5% of all newborns to a fraction of this figure."[17]

Medical, pharmaceutical and health professionals were trained at higher, intermediate and basic levels to meet the demands. The number of medical and pharmaceutical colleges and schools, short-term training programs, intermediate medical schools and training classes doubled in a year from 1949 to 1950, and they continued to grow in the following years. Enrollment of students increased 176.5 percent in 1950 over 1949, and 142.9 percent in 1952 over 1951. Students at medical colleges in 1950 and 1951 were 60 percent more than the total number of doctors trained in the past seven decades.[18] However, the low literacy rate of the Chinese population, at about 15 percent at the time, seriously hampered health reconstruction as well as every other aspect of economic and social development. To tackle the problem, a nationwide anti-illiteracy movement was launched immediately after the founding of the PRC, which significantly reduced the illiteracy rate in the decades of the 1950s and 1960s. By 1964, the literacy rate increased to 63 percent of the population.[19]

Building health organizations and facilities at the basic level was carried out simultaneously with the expansion of health personnel. "The Decision to Fully Build and Develop Health Organizations at the Basic Level in the Entire Country" was adopted at the National Health Conference in 1950. The decision specified that every city district and every rural village must have a medical and health unit. Rural health organizations included county people's hospitals as the main medical institution, subdistrict/town health stations, administrative village health committees, and health workers of natural villages or hamlets. They formed a tiered rural health structure in parallel to local government administration. By the end of 1952, China had 2,102 county hospitals and 7,961 subdistrict health stations established, covering more than 90 percent of all counties.[20] District health stations and village health organizations adopted diverse forms of medical practices, with some government-run and others government–private jointly run. United clinics or medical cooperatives were also organized with government subsidies.[21]

Following the Soviet model of disease prevention, China established the Health and Epidemic Prevention Stations at the county level in the early 1950s to direct the work of local disease control and prevention. The station was a comprehensive technical agency that dealt with all aspects of disease prevention, vaccination, health education and research, and public health campaigns to align with national health and economic development. The Health and Epidemic Prevention Stations formed a national disease-prevention infrastructure that characterized China's anti-epidemic disease programs. The station was gradually expanded into subdistricts and rural towns. By 1957, China had established 1,626 epidemic prevention stations that covered more than two thirds of all counties, along with other specialized centers for the control of specific diseases such as malaria, tuberculosis, schistosomiasis, brucellosis, and other diseases. In 1985, the number of epidemic prevention stations increased to 3,410 with a total staff of 144,998.[22] The Ministry of Health continuously updated the "Rules of the Work of the Health and Epidemic Prevention Stations" from 1954 to adjust to new needs and approaches. The regular modifications of rules demonstrated that Chinese health workers constantly drew lessons from their experience to improve the methods of disease control and prevention.

Factories, mining districts, and railways organized their own basic health units and medical services that were operated by their safety and health protection committees. As a result, injuries and occupational disease rates of workers and staff fell from 6.4 percent in 1949 to 1.6 percent in 1951.[23] Additionally, numerous teams of epidemic prevention and medical services were dispatched to serve the millions who were working on large projects, such as the harnessing of Huai River, the dredging of Yi River, the flood diversion of Qing River, and the construction of the Chengdu–Chongqing railway line.

Their health work ensured no outbreaks of epidemics and the successful completion of those large projects. In June 1952, the State Council issued a directive that free medical care was to be offered to all government workers and members of political parties and organizations.[24] Free medical care was gradually extended to other groups in the following years.

In 1952, news media increasingly reported American use of germ warfare against China and North Korea in the Korean War. The alleged American germ warfare caused anxiety and anger among the Chinese people. The fear of biological warfare added new implications to national security and health campaigns.[25] Chinese leaders called on the people to combine health protection of the people with the defense of the motherland. The whole country was mobilized to launch sanitary and hygiene campaigns to clean up communities and kill bugs to defeat American germ warfare and imperialism. People participated with patriotic enthusiasm in the cleaning up and the elimination of flies and mosquitoes. The popular slogan was "Killing one housefly is equivalent to destroying one American imperialist."[26] Hundreds of thousands of people attended political rallies against germ warfare, with demands for international justice against American war crimes. The health movement rallied people to unite against enemies and diseases, which newspapers hailed as the Great Patriotic Health Movement. The campaigns against germ warfare during the Korean War shaped the national health principle of combining the mass movement with health work. The Patriotic Mass Health Movement became thereafter an annual health campaign across China up to the 1980s.

The Political and Social Meanings of People's Health

When the Second National Health Conference was held in late 1952, Chairman Mao Zedong sent his instruction: "Mobilize the people to pay attention to hygiene and reduce diseases, improve the people's health to smash the enemy's germ warfare."[27] Mao's instruction significantly encouraged the Great Patriotic Health Movement. Political activists and health organizers immediately started to mobilize people with "eight cleans" (clean children, bodies, interior of homes, courtyards, streets and lanes, kitchens, toilets, and pigsties), "five kills" (kill flies, mosquitoes, lice, fleas, and bedbugs) and "one catch" (catch rats). Across China, people young and old learned the rudimentary of public health and took action to improve environmental sanitation and personal hygiene. Garbage was removed, sewage lines and drainage systems cleared and restored, and dirty water pools and ponds filled up. The health movement aimed to utilize people's power and science to tackle sanitation problems and personal hygiene for disease prevention and public health. It turned the masses from passive recipients of health services into active agents to detect and fight diseases. Scholars used the term *mass mobilization model* to characterize Chinese health campaigns from the 1950s to the 1980s.[28]

The anti-disease campaigns energized national patriotic enthusiasm to defend the motherland and defeat American imperialism. For the hundreds of millions of Chinese people, participation in the movement was a personal contribution to national defense and health improvement of socialist reconstruction.[29] They were eager to learn scientific knowledge about improving health to increase production and become cultured persons. The popular slogan was "to transform social traditions and re-create the world." In cities, health campaigns were organized by work units and neighborhood committees for routine cleaning activities to make their place nice and clean as a civilized unit. In rural countryside, health campaigns were combined with land reclamation and irrigation construction and emphasized the improvement of sanitary conditions for humans and livestock. Media and public events promoted the people's health as an important part of the socialist reconstruction of China, where the well-being of people was emphasized in contrast to the exploitation of people in a capitalist system. The health movement showcased the political significance of the Chinese socialist revolution and the discourse of the superiority of socialism over capitalism.

The central government made disease prevention and the people's health part of the state planning of economic growth and national development. Following the Soviet model, the Chinese government created state planning to guide national economic development and reconstruction. In the first Five-Year Plan (1953–1957), Chinese leaders outlined the construction of a socialist society with new health programs and services to demonstrate the long-term commitment to people's health as a national priority. The five-year plan stated that as industrial production progressed, factories would provide labor insurance and health protection, government employees would have free medical care, and health facilities would be strengthened to protect people's health in cities and countryside. The government policies were widely disseminated via media and popular health education material. The Shanghai Anti-Tuberculosis Association printed national health policies and programs at the very beginning of a series of anti-tuberculosis posters in 1954.[30] People's health was not only fundamental to the well-being of individuals but also important to national economic productivity, national defense, and social transformation. Chinese policy-makers were acutely aware of the social and economic drains caused by epidemic diseases and natural disasters when they deliberated on the guidelines of national development.

Political discourse reinforced the central idea that Chinese people were now masters of their own country under the leadership of the Chinese Communist Party and that they were learning socialist ideas and playing active roles in building a socialist China. Millions of peasants, workers, and soldiers attended literacy classes in the evenings after work. They learned to read and write and studied government laws and policies, scientific knowledge of industrial and agricultural production, and knowledge about epidemic diseases—all the things directly related to their daily life. In rural China, where the illiteracy rate was much higher than in cities and traditional views were strong with widespread epidemic diseases, farmers learned to read and write to empower themselves with modern scientific knowledge of agriculture and disease prevention for livestock.[31] Literacy proved key to transforming people's old mentality and reshaping their new attitude and behavior. From 1949 to 1956, approximately 294 million Chinese people attended literacy classes, with the majority being peasants, and 20.76 million got rid of illiteracy.[32] Illiteracy rate in China dropped from 85 percent in 1949 to 37 percent in 1964.[33]

The dissemination of scientific knowledge of disease popularized germ theory and strengthened the concept of "scientific medicine." Visual materials such as posters, pictorials, charts, pictures, bulletins, and wallpapers were popular with ordinary people because visual images helped them understand what germs looked like and how flies and mosquitoes spread diseases.[34] People wanted to hear vivid stories and learn things they could use in daily life. In rural health education, farmers were more interested in learning how to deal with head scratches and bleeding than CPR (cardiopulmonary resuscitation) first aid because head scratches and bleedings were much more common than CPR. To make scientific knowledge accessible to ordinary people, health workers used simple and colloquial language to write and popularize scientific concepts and subjects.[35]

Health campaigns changed people more broadly than merely conveying information about disease prevention and health improvement. Public health programs generated social changes as they drove home the social and political meanings of health in the transformation of individual citizens and society. China's social approach to disease prevention, in addition to the mass vaccination, addressed the socioeconomic causes of disease and changed people's traditional view of fatalism to an active can-do attitude. It reshaped their behavior with the social and cultural expectations of the socialist citizenry. Hygienic behavior was praised as a civilized way of life that people were encouraged to develop to become respected citizens. Health advocacy emphasized not only the strong physique but the mental and spiritual health of citizens as well. Personal cleanliness and tidiness were promoted along with public hygiene. Individuals' health and health behavior was viewed as part of a community improvement that benefited the society at large. Health education materials highlighted the collective action of people working together to fight diseases by dredging rivers and filling up ditches.[36] In the sanitary and hygienic campaigns, cities, communities, workplaces and schools competed for the best results and the titles of "civilized communities" and "civilized persons."

In the anti-tuberculosis campaigns, the hygienic behavior of not spitting was particularly highlighted as a civilized virtue. Spitting was described as a dangerous behavior that caused the spread of tuberculosis. It was criticized as an uncivilized behavior that was socially and culturally unacceptable. People were instructed to spit into a spittoon or a handkerchief if they had to. Tuberculosis used to carry the social stigma of death, spitting now signified a person's barbaric and uncivilized traits. A model citizen in socialist China was expected to be healthy, clean and civilized. Signs of "Do not spit on the ground! Splitting is uncivilized!" were displayed in parks, public spaces, and at workplaces and schools. The omnipresent fixation on anti-spitting was, in fact, not unique to China but quite universal in all countries' anti-tuberculosis programs. In the early 20th-century United States, for example, the anti-tuberculosis movement demonstrated similar zeal against spitting as an immoral and barbaric behavior. It gained a serious moral stake in health awakening that helped spread the germ theory among Americans.[37] The anti-spitting advocacy in China's tuberculosis prevention shaped people's health and hygienic views and behavior with socialist moral virtues.

From the Soviet Model to Self-Reliance: Urban and Rural Healthcare and the Barefoot Doctors

The Soviet Union had a significant but short-term influence on China's socialist reconstruction in the 1950s. The people's health applied Soviet concepts and methods to Chinese circumstances. The institutional system of people's health relied on a diverse structure of comprehensive hospitals, hospitals of Chinese medicine, hospitals for infectious diseases, health and epidemic prevention stations, women's and children's health institutes, community health clinics, and other institutions. Numerous hospitals and clinics were built to provide state-run medical services to the people after the transition from private to organized medical practice in the early 1950s. The Health Ministry issued "Provisional Regulations on the Management of Hospitals and Clinics" and the "Decision on Strengthening and Developing the Basic-Level Health Organizations" in 1951 and the "General Rules for the Organization of County Hospitals" in 1952 to strengthen healthcare services at the basic level, particularly in the county (*xian*) and rural countryside, where more than 80 percent of the Chinese population lived.[38] Those policy measures standardized the organization and operation of hospitals and clinics across the country and guided the development of healthcare with a significant extension of services to rural and remote places. As hospitals and clinics became state-run institutions, although certain forms of private practice continued during the transitional 1950s, China moved toward a free healthcare system with socialist aspirations. The government invested heavily in building comprehensive hospitals as the main medical institutions for people's health. Comprehensive hospitals, which constituted more than 90 percent of all hospitals in China, were general hospitals that treated all kinds of diseases. They provided preventive services and lent professional expertise to local and industrial health campaigns as well. Urban districts established basic-level health stations and clinics to provide rudimentary medical services and disease prevention. Factories and companies established their own hospitals and clinics, following the Soviet model. A hierarchical structure of the hospital system gradually took shape, despite the fact they were all called the people's hospitals, with the best doctors working at top hospitals usually designated as the provincial or municipal hospitals. The second tier was at the prefectural or city level, and the third tier at the county level.

The county hospitals, although at the lower end of the urban comprehensive hospital structure, occupied a uniquely important place in the chain of urban and rural healthcare system because they were the main medical institutions in counties that provided technical guidance and support to rural health institutions in towns and villages. Rural healthcare networks developed during the different phases of agricultural collectivization, with the formation of a three-tiered rural health system composed of the county hospital, the town hospital station, and the village medical office. The 1949–1955 period saw land reforms and mutual aid in the agriculture sector when land was distributed among peasants and medical services shifted from private to organized practice of united clinics. Medical practitioners and traditional healers were encouraged to join local medical workers' associations and form united clinics. Those who wished to continue practicing medicine by themselves were allowed to do so by the government. In the high stage of collective farming when the people's communes were organized in the latter half of the 1950s, commune-sponsored medical cooperatives replaced the united clinics to provide healthcare for farmers. The county hospital became the leading force in promoting modern medicine and public health in the rural communes of the entire county.

In cities, doctors of Western medicine and traditional Chinese medicine formed their own united hospitals and clinics in the early 1950s. Flexible government policies led to diverse types of medical practice in the early stage of socialist reconstruction. The organized medical practice of united hospitals and clinics, nonetheless, changed the operation of medical service. Doctors became cooperative partners of the government in providing healthcare to the people, even though they ran the operation of their own united clinics. They also promoted and participated in anti-epidemic disease campaigns as medical professionals. The united hospitals and clinics were the initial step of transforming private medical practice into organized healthcare under the government's auspices, in parallel to the economic transition from private enterprises to national enterprises.

Hospitals and clinics became state-run when China embarked on the road of socialist reconstruction after the Korean War. In 1953, the government restructured the national system of administration with provinces, municipalities, and autonomous regions under the central government. Health departments, bureaus, and offices were established at every level of province, prefecture, municipality, city, county, and town, making a national system of health administration under the Ministry of Health. With the influence of the Soviet Union, China restructured the medical education system to shorten medical colleges from eight to five years. There were about 50,000 doctors of Western medicine in 1950, and more than 100,000 new doctors of Western medicine were trained between 1950 and 1966, which was a major achievement in terms of producing doctors. China's large population, however, made the doctor-to-patient ratio far below the standard of advanced nations. Health leaders used a variety of methods to alleviate the pressure by training large numbers of health professionals via short-term programs of different levels, paying particular attention to the urgent need for basic-level health workers and maternal nurses.[39]

In addition to doctors of Western medicine, China had more than 500,000 doctors of Chinese medicine in 1950. Most of them practiced medicine in rural towns. The Health Ministry, however, disqualified large numbers of them between 1949 and 1952 by using biased examinations in the name of upholding the scientific standards of medicine. The discrimination and marginalization of Chinese medicine and its practitioners significantly disrupted health services in rural towns and caused widespread resentment among the people. Political leaders of the central government also became concerned about the situation. When the Central Political Bureau discussed national health work in November 1953, Chairman Mao Zedong emphasized the value of Chinese medicine: "China has made great contributions to the world, Chinese medicine being one of them … Chinese and Western medicine must unite."[40] Mao's speech brought changes in the policy of the Health Ministry toward Chinese medicine. Thereafter, doctors of Chinese medicine were allowed to work in hospitals to provide a variety of health services and the use of Chinese drugs. For the first time, doctors of Chinese medicine were admitted to the Chinese Medical Association as members. Moreover, colleges and hospitals of Chinese medicine, and the China Academy of Chinese Medical Sciences were established. Doctors of Western and Chinese medicine were encouraged to learn from each other to enrich their medical knowledge and broaden their ability to diagnose and treat illnesses. In the mutual learning of Chinese and Western medicine, a third type of medicine emerged, which was called integrated medicine (中成药). Tu Youyou (屠呦呦, 1930–), who won the Nobel Prize in Medicine in 2015, was a student of both Western and Chinese medicine. She exemplified the success of combining the age-old Chinese medicine with the modern biomedicine. She started as a student of Western biomedicine at the Medical College of Beijing University in the 1950s. Upon graduation, she began working at the China Academy of Chinese Medicine. Tu studied Chinese medicine and pharmacology at the Academy and applied biomedical research and analysis to the study of Chinese medicine. It was this integration of biomedical research with Chinese medicine that led Tu's team of medical scientists to the successful extraction of artemisinin from a plant of traditional Chinese medicine to make an effective malaria drug. Artemisinin has saved millions of lives in the world since its extraction in the early 1970s.

In the anti-disease campaigns, China was influenced by the Soviet methods of using epidemic prevention centers to direct local disease prevention. China created a national network of epidemic prevention stations to coordinate national campaigns of disease prevention and health communication, as discussed in the previous section. In tuberculosis prevention, for instance, China followed the Soviet model by setting up tuberculosis hospitals and sanatoria as centers of treatment and recovery. Factories and mining companies established sanatoria and resting rooms for tuberculosis patients. Railway Labor Unions organized their own sanatoria with each having a staff of tuberculosis health specialists and 150–200 beds.[41] Sanatoria admitted people of less acute conditions and helped them recover in a relaxed and pleasant environment with lots of fresh air, sunshine, nutritious food and good rest. The goal was to help the patients recover so that they would return as healthy and productive workers.[42] The anti-tuberculosis campaigns concentrated on the protection of children and workers in factories and mines where the incidence of the disease was high. People were given the BCG (Bacille Calmette-Guérin) vaccine and screened with X-rays. Mobile medical teams brought the BCG vaccines to factories, schools, and urban and rural communities. Health education instructed people not to spit on the ground, to maintain sanitation and personal hygiene, and to keep healthy habits such as sleeping well, eating nutritious food, doing exercises, and opening windows for fresh air. Those preventive measures were quite similar to the anti-tuberculosis programs in many postwar countries where the BCG vaccine and X-ray checkups were used for children and adults. In China, after years of coordinated measures of comprehensive prevention and improvement of food nutrition, the tuberculosis incidence dropped from 4 percent in 1950 to 1.5 percent in 1965, while the mortality rate declined from 280 to 40 per 100,000 in the same period.[43]

Soviet science, especially Pavlov's theory, impacted Chinese science and the scientization of Chinese medicine in the 1950s. Chinese intellectuals updated themselves with the latest Soviet scientific research and theories while they were politically reeducated to be "red and expert."[44] Soviet research was increasingly translated and published in Chinese medical journals. The most celebrated successful application of Pavlov's theory was the scientific theorization of Chinese acupuncture, called the *New Acupuncture* (新针灸学).[45] Soviet influence was noticeable in many other areas beyond health, such as arts and culture, science and education, and industries. Thousands of Soviet professional experts and technicians worked in China. In the late 1950s, however, Sino–Soviet relations appeared strained. After Nikita S. Khrushchev became the Soviet leader, he started a campaign of de-Stalinization with major policy changes. His personal attacks on Stalin and his policy of peaceful coexistence with the capitalist West made Chinese leaders uneasy. Disagreements increased between China and the Soviet Union when Khrushchev openly criticized China's domestic programs and undermined China's position in international affairs. In 1960, the Soviet Union decided to stop aiding China by calling back home technicians while pressuring China to pay back loans. China suffered significantly with hundreds of major contracts canceled and ongoing technical projects abandoned, including an atomic-bomb construction project.

The movement to learn from the Soviet Union came to an end when Sino-Soviet relations deteriorated into an open hostility in the early 1960s. The two big communist countries, thereafter, engaged in a long and heated ideological debate on what was true communism. China opposed the hegemony of both the United States and the Soviet Union with strong political rhetoric of self-reliance and independence in building socialism. In fact, China had been carving out its own road of socialist reconstruction long before the split with the Soviet Union. The second Five-Year Plan of 1957 showed that Chinese leaders made adjustments to national economic plans by balancing out light and heavy industries and accelerating the collectivization of the agricultural sector, apparently with the aim to reduce its reliance on the Soviet Union. In terms of disease prevention and health reconstruction, the national program of agricultural development of 1956 made clear that China aimed to achieve basic eradication of the diseases that severely harmed the people, such as malaria, schistosomiasis, and so on. In the same year, a national conference was held to discuss specific guidelines and measures to eradicate malaria within seven years.[46] Although China did not eradicate malaria in seven years, it made significant progress in reducing and controlling malaria. Cases of malaria declined from 102.8 per 10,000 in 1955 to 21.6 per 10,000 in 1958, a drop of 80 percent. The anti-malaria campaigns were coordinated in the national Patriotic Health Movement against all diseases, but specific preventive measures were taken to tackle particular diseases such as malaria. In the early 1960s and early 1970s, respectively, malaria made a comeback with widespread outbreaks, when the country suffered economic failures in the wake of the Great Leap Forward, and then the political turmoil with large population movement across cities in the early stage of the Cultural Revolution. Malaria incidence was finally brought down in 1982 to the level of 1959, thanks to years of strenuous efforts and the new effective drug made with artemisinin. China achieved basic control of malaria in the early 1990s and declared the eradication of malaria in 2021.[47]

The Great Leap Forward, which was a movement to accelerate national economy and social advancement, clearly demonstrated Chinese leaders' desire to make China strong with an independent road of development in the face of increasing tensions with the Soviet Union. Launched in 1958 to speed up industrial and agricultural modernization, the movement integrated people's health in the national socioeconomic advancement. When the organization of people's communes accelerated and reshaped agricultural production and rural administration, collective medical services for farmers were increasingly sponsored by the commune's funds. The Health Ministry supported the organization of people's commune's collective healthcare, but it cautioned about over-enthusiasm. It instructed that well-off communes could experiment with collective healthcare, but communes that had been using self-sponsored medical care did not need to rush to collective healthcare. The ministry expected the people's communes to develop collective healthcare gradually according to the level of production and people's willingness to join. The pay for collective healthcare workers was expected to be no less than their pre-commune level. Despite the Health Ministry's cautious guidance, an enthusiastic wave to form commune-sponsored healthcare swept across the country.[48] No communes would like to be left behind in the high time of collectivization.[49]

When the agricultural sector suffered major setbacks in the three years following the 1958 Great Leap Forward, many communes could not sustain the expenses of collective healthcare. As a result, rural medical services declined. By 1964, only about 30 percent of communes and production brigades continued to operate medical cooperatives.[50] At the same time, the majority of college-trained medical personnel stayed in city hospitals including county hospitals. Few went to work in commune hospitals or rural health stations. Data from 1964 showed that 69 percent of college-trained (high-level) medical personnel worked in cities and 31 percent in counties, including 10 percent in rural communes. Among the health school–trained (intermediate-level) medical personnel, 57 percent were in cities and 43 percent in counties, including 27 percent in rural communes. The majority of medical workers in rural China continued to be practitioners of traditional Chinese medicine, even though the newly trained local health workers had been filling up the ranks. In terms of medical expenditure, 30 percent of the national health budget was spent on free healthcare for state employees, whereas 27 percent was spent on the countryside including counties, and 16 percent on rural population in the communes.[51] Apparently, the highly trained medical doctors tended to stay in cities while the intermediate level health personnel tended to work in county and commune hospitals. This professional divergence contributed to the institutional hierarchy of quality medical services. Moreover, two types of healthcare coexisted in China as the health system developed. One was the state-sponsored free healthcare for state employees mostly in cities, and the other was the commune-sponsored collective healthcare in rural communes that were of inferior benefits than the state-sponsored healthcare.[52]

The 1964 data revealed a huge gap between urban and rural access to medical services and health protection. Political leaders noticed the problem when they read about the health situation. In a significant move to redirect health work in China and an obvious criticism of the Health Ministry, Chairman Mao Zedong called on the country to "put the emphasis of health work in the countryside." The major newspaper, *The People's Daily*, published Mao's call with editorial advocacy on June 26, 1965. Known thereafter as the June 26 instruction, Mao's call had a huge impact on the new development of rural health in the following decade when the political movement of the Cultural Revolution attacked bourgeois thought and emphasized serving the people. A new type of rural doctor emerged during the Cultural Revolution, who was called the barefoot doctor.

Some argued that Mao's attention to rural health was influenced by his concerns over national security, as the Soviet Union and the United States both put pressures on China at the time.[53] Mao openly criticized the Health

Ministry at the Third People's Congress in January 1965. He complained that medical education took too long to produce doctors. After Mao's complaint, leaders of the central government immediately started working with the Health Ministry with specific instructions on how to improve rural health work.[54] Changes came quickly in medical education when the Health Ministry added three-year programs to the existing medical education and increased student enrollments to produce more doctors for the countryside. The Health Ministry aimed to achieve the goal of staffing each production brigade with a midwife and each production team with a health worker within the next three to five years.[55] Mobile medical teams of city doctors were sent to rural areas on a regular basis with prominent physicians on the teams to provide training to local health workers and offer treatment for severe illnesses. By April 1965, more than 1,520 mobile medical teams of 18,600 doctors were already in the countryside. But it was too small a number to make a significant difference in rural healthcare, as hundreds of millions of farmers needed medical services. It is important to note that 80 percent of the 715 million Chinese population lived in rural China in 1965. The Health Ministry proposed to reduce medical college education from six to five years and pharmacy college training from five to four years in August 1965. Meanwhile, more educated rural youth were recruited and trained as part-time health workers and midwives to serve their fellow villagers. Those part-time health workers participated in farming work while providing rudimentary health services in the field. Their work was mainly compensated with work points and, therefore, cost little extra to the commune and production brigade in which they worked.

The part-time health workers were highly popular with farmers because they came from them and provided them immediate attention when they became sick. Farmers called the part-time rural health workers "barefoot doctors" because they worked in the rice paddies bare-footed just like the farmers they served. "Barefoot doctor" was an endearment that the farmers gave to the health worker. When the Cultural Revolution (1966–1976) began, the training of barefoot doctors gained momentum with the enthusiasm of implementing Mao's June 26 instruction and addressing the unequal access to healthcare between cities and the countryside. A new wave of developing medical cooperatives in the people's communes and production brigades took hold of the country again. Rural medical cooperatives were celebrated as a new socialist creation that brought medical services to the people.

There was a transfer of medical resources from cities to the countryside during the Cultural Revolution. Doctors, professionals and urban youth were sent down to rural communes for re-education. The sent-down professionals, due to their high level of education and expertise, were immediately put to work as doctors and teachers in the communes and production brigades instead of working in the field. The sent-down doctors were placed to work in county and commune hospitals, where the quality of medical care was consequently strengthened. They trained rural youths as barefoot doctors to work in production brigades and teams. The training concentrated on three major areas: (1) knowledge about twenty to thirty types of the most common local diseases, treatment of minor illnesses and injuries, use of simple first aid, prescription of commonly used drugs, and basic methods of acupuncture; (2) knowledge of how to eliminate the four pests, how to provide hygienic treatment of water and waste, and how to carry out the patriotic health movement and health education; and (3) knowledge of how to report epidemics and use simple methods to prevent contagious diseases such as the vaccination injection. Training of rural midwives emphasized the ability to use new delivery methods, carry out prenatal examinations, provide care for the puerperal mother and baby, and conduct family planning education.[56] Training time varied from short courses of a few months to a year at commune and county hospitals, with follow-up advanced training and internship at different levels. The goal was to teach them knowledge of prevention and treatment of the most common epidemic and endemic diseases with both Chinese and Western medicine. Their study was usually tailored to local conditions, with an emphasis on combining Chinese and Western medicine and relying on local resources. The specific requirements for rural health workers and midwives provided a standard of basic health service in rural China, although the quality varied depending on the capability of individuals and the availability of local resources and support. Barefoot doctors were able to provide independent curative and preventive treatment, even providing basic prescriptions for drugs. Their services made farmers' life significantly convenient when they needed immediate medical help. Without barefoot doctors, farmers had to travel long hours to commune and county hospitals, which meant the loss of work plus travel expenses. Economic factors usually deterred people from seeking medical help from afar.

Barefoot doctors were paramedics in rural China. They often worked with mobile medical teams to provide medical treatment and learn new techniques. They referred patients to commune and county hospitals when the illnesses were beyond their professional capability. In the prevention of acute epidemic diseases such as malaria and schistosomiasis, they took blood samples and provided timely treatment. They encouraged people to report sick cases to health workers for immediate treatment and prevention. They also led people in rural health campaigns to dig wells for clean water and build sanitary toilets, pigsties and animal sheds. Farmers were instructed to change wood stoves into chimney stoves and enlarge windows to keep the kitchens clean and bright and well ventilated. Rural sanitary movements concentrated on "two managements and five improvements"—management of water and waste, and improvement of latrines, animal sheds, wells, stoves, and home environment. Sanitation and health improvement were promoted as the modern transformation of the countryside. Farmers would follow the instructions when they sensed it economically beneficial, but many a time, barefoot doctors had to educate them the importance of health with political significance.

Barefoot doctors were hailed as the new phenomenon of socialism, who served the people with warmth and improved rural health. Political qualifications were emphasized for the barefoot doctors during the Cultural Revolution. They were expected to be born into a good family like a poor peasant family with revolutionary enthusiasm, loving rural China and willing to serve the people wholeheartedly. It was considered a honor to become a barefoot doctor personally, and the position brought pride to the family. Female barefoot doctors gained particular attention, as government policies promoted gender equality. Women were encouraged to achieve what men did with the slogan of "women can hold half of the sky." Women were projected as the public image of health profession in socialist China, a demonstration of women's liberation from past oppression. There were, however, more female doctors in cities than in the countryside. The majority of rural parents still held the traditional ideas of schooling their sons rather than their daughters, despite the government's persistent efforts to transform people's thoughts from the old to the new. Among the barefoot doctors, about one third were female due to lack of educated rural females for the job. Some sent-down youths were recruited and trained as barefoot doctors when no local youths were qualified. By the end of 1975, China had more than 1.5 million barefoot doctors and another 3.9 million health technicians and midwives working directly for farmers in production brigades and teams. More than 65 percent of the national health budget was spent on the rural population, where hospital beds increased from 40 percent to 60 percent of the national total from 1965 to 1975.[57] By 1980, over 90 percent of production brigades had established medical cooperatives to provide healthcare for 85 percent of the rural population.[58] Those positive developments were remarkable in an otherwise destructive era of the Cultural Revolution. The growth of medical cooperatives and the increase of barefoot doctors mutually influenced each other in the provision of rural collective healthcare. They were both dependent on the collective agricultural system of the people's communes.[59]

Conclusion

The socialist health reconstruction of China was significantly affected by the superpowers' rivalry in shaping the post–World War II world order. The United States' isolation of China with economic sanctions and military threats in the Cold War only edged China further toward the Soviet Union for economic aid and political and military support. Although China followed the Soviet model in socialist modernization in the 1950s, its policies and programs demonstrated a significant Chinese tendency for independence and self-reliance. The people's health, which meant not only the health protection of people but also the foundation for a healthy workforce for national economic development, was fully integrated in the state planning of socioeconomic reconstruction of a strong and prosperous China. It was advocated as a long-term commitment of the state to the people in building a just and equal society, even though the result was less than the promise. In the national health campaigns, health matters were not merely medical concerns but political issues in the socioeconomic transformation of the society.

Anti-disease campaigns were characterized with the social and political mobilization of the masses for hygiene, disease detection and report, and vaccination. The coordination and collaboration across administrative departments and sectors with active community participation proved effective in controlling and eradicating the epidemic diseases that had been plaguing tens of millions of Chinese. In the meantime, health work acted as a force of sociopolitical transformation of the people in getting rid of old habits and cultivating new attitudes about disease and health behavior. Citizens in socialist China were expected to have civilized behavior of hygiene, while the people's health was hailed as the demonstration of socialist superiority over capitalism. Health communication used visual images to disseminate scientific information about germs and diseases to modernize people's scientific knowledge of health and to empower them to become active fighters against diseases instead of passive recipients of medical services. It should be noted that people did not automatically become active in the health movement. There was reluctance and resistance to the campaigns because health work took time and effort that required resources and commitment. Moreover, health work challenged traditional views and lifestyles that people were reluctant to change.

The process of China's health reconstruction illuminated the transformation of the society when anti-disease campaigns were incorporated in the overall sociopolitical and economic modernization. After the initial transition from private to organized medical practice, state-run hospitals and clinics provided medical and health services in cities, while commune-sponsored medical cooperatives were established to provide medical and health services in rural communes. China's socialist healthcare system developed in parallel with its industrial nationalization and agricultural collectivization that transformed China from the old to the new. Health work was guided by socialist ideology and patriotic enthusiasm to serve the people.

The most remarkable change in China's healthcare, which was very different from the Soviet Union, was the creation of health services in the rural countryside. China advocated self-reliance in socialist reconstruction after relations with the Soviet Union deteriorated. The three-tiered rural healthcare network, together with the construction of medical cooperatives and the training of barefoot doctors, made medical services available to the huge rural population. Barefoot doctors played a vital role in rural healthcare. At the peak time of collective rural healthcare in 1978, about 5 million barefoot doctors and midwives provided basic health services to about 800 million rural population. The quality of health service, however, varied significantly from place to place, due to local economic resources, technical equipment availability, the professional level of health workers, and local bureaucracy.[60] Given the challenging situation of a large population and limited access to international technical advancement during the Cold War, Chinese health leaders pragmatically prioritized the number of health workers in building the people's health. In the 1980s' economic reforms when the agricultural sector underwent a fundamental change from the commune system to the household responsible system, rural medical cooperatives collapsed, and barefoot doctors could not function any more due to the loss of the supporting system that had sustained them. At the same time, Chinese health leaders turned their attention to medical technology to pursue efficiency and profits in increasingly market-oriented medical care.

The institutional infrastructure of the people's health relied on the state-sponsored hospital system that contained a variety of hospitals, institutes, clinics, and stations at different levels of the province, municipality, city, county, and rural town. Different from the Soviet Union, China promoted its traditional medical knowledge with an emphasis on combining Western and Chinese medicine and the scientization of Chinese medicine. Those health policies helped enrich the medical and health resources for the people's health. They even led to the development of a third type of medicine called integrated medicine in China. As the national healthcare system developed, a parallel of two healthcare structures emerged with people of state-owned enterprises enjoying state-sponsored healthcare, while people of collective-owned enterprises, which included all rural communities and some urban and rural business enterprises, enjoying collective-sponsored healthcare. The benefits of state-sponsored health programs outnumbered that of collective-sponsored health programs. The divergence between urban and rural healthcare became clear when rural China lacked well-trained medical personnel and resources. Despite the low level of healthcare in many rural communes, the availability of medical and health services by barefoot doctors and midwives made a huge difference to the lives of hundreds of millions of people in rural China. The population increased from 600 million to 981 million between 1950 and 1980. Life expectancy increased from 38 to 60 between 1949 and 1965 and from 60 to 68 between 1965 and 1980, due to the eradication and control of diseases, available health services, and the increase of general living standards.[61]

Notes

1 "Two Health Ministries Instruct the Launch of Military and Civilian Spring Campaigns against Epidemic Diseases," *The People's Daily*, February 11, 1950. The two health ministries were the health ministry of the military and the health ministry of the government. Mainland China was divided into six military regions for governance during 1949–1952 when the country was recovering from war devastation to normal functions of socio-economic life.
2 *30 Years' Review of China's Science and Technology, 1949–1979* (Singapore: World Scientific, 1981). Thomas P. Bernstein and Hua-Yu Li, eds., *China Learns from the Soviet Union, 1949-Present* (Lexington Books, 2011). History of Science and Technology in the People's Republic of China, Wikipedia, accessed August 22, 2021.

https://en.wikipedia.org/wiki/History_of_science_and_technology_in_the_People%27s_Republic_of_China.

3 Gao Xi, "Foreign Models of Medicine in Twentieth-Century China," in *Medical Transitions in Twentieth-Century China*, eds. Bridie Andrews and Mary Brown Bullock (Bloomington: Indiana University Press, 2014).

4 David M. Lampton, "Public Health and Politics in China's Past Two Decades," *Health Services Reports* 87, no. 10 (December 1972): 896.

5 Liming Lee, "The Current State of Public Health in China," *Annual Review of Public Health* 25 (2004): 327–28.

6 Chen Haifeng, *Zhongguo weisheng baojian shi* [History of Healthcare in China] (Shanghai: Shanghai kexue jishu chubanshe, 1992), 81.

7 For the continuity of practices and principles, see Liping Bu, *Public Health and the Modernization of China, 1865–2015* (London: Routledge, 2017), chapters 3 and 4.

8 Li Teh-chuan, "The People's Health Services" in *Culture, Education and Health in New China* (Peking: Foreign Language Press, 1952), 38–39.

9 Qu Wanlin, "Guancha xin Zhongguo de yige shijiao—shixi Longxugou zhili yu xin Zhongguo xingxiang [A Perspective of Observing the New China: An Analysis of the Transformation of Longxugou and the Image of New China]," *Dangdai Zhongguo shi yanjiu* [Historical Studies of Contemporary China] 14.2 (March 2007): 46–51.

10 The famous Chinese playwright, Lao She, wrote a play called *Long Xu Gou* (Dragon Beard Ditch, 1951) to illuminate the fundamental transformation of the place and the people in his hometown of Beijing.

11 For a historical study of vaccination in China, see Mary Augusta Brazelton, *Mass Vaccination: Citizens' Bodies and State Power in Modern China* (Cornell: Cornell University Press, 2019).

12 Li Teh-chuan, "The People's Health Services," 31.

13 Xingjian Xu, "Control of Communicable Diseases in the People's Republic of China," *Asia Pacific Journal of Public Health* 7, no. 2 (1994): 123–131.

14 Li Teh-chuan, "The People's Health Services," 32.

15 Weishengbu jicheng weisheng he fuyou baojian si [Bureau of Basic Health and the Women's and Children's Health of the Ministry of Health], *Nongcun weisheng wenjian huibian (1951–2000)* [Collections of Documents on Rural Health Work, 1951–2000] (Ministry of Health, PRC, 2001), pp. 247–248.

16 Ibid.

17 David Hipgrave, "Communicable Disease Control in China: From Mao to Now," *Journal of Global Health* 1, no. 2 (December 2011): 226.

18 Li Teh-chuan, "The People's Health Services," 36.

19 Yu Bo and Xie Guodong, *Zhongguo saomang jiaoyu* [Literacy Education in China] (Harbin: Dongbei linye daxue chubanshe, 1998).

20 Chen Haifeng, *Zhongguo weisheng baojian shi*, 90.

21 For united clinics or medical cooperatives in the early 1950s, see Xiaoping Fang, *Barefoot Doctors and Western Medicine in China* (New York: University of Rochester Press, 2012).

22 David Hipgrave, "Communicable Disease Control in China: From Mao to Now," 225; and Chen Haifeng, *Zhongguo weisheng baojian shi*, 109.

23 Li Teh-chuan, "The People's Health Services," 34.

24 Ibid., 34–35.

25 Different perspectives on the germ warfare include Yang Nianqun, "Disease Prevention, Social Mobilization and Spatial Politics: The Anti-Germ Warfare Incident of 1952 and the 'Patriotic Health Campaign,'" *The Chinese Historical Review* 11, no. 2 (2004): 155–182; Ruth Rogaski, "Nature, Annihilation, and Modernity: China's Korean War Germ-Warfare Experience Reconsidered," *Journal of Asian Studies* 61, no. 2 (2002): 381–415; and Stephen Endicott and Edward Hageman,

The United States and Biological Warfare: Secrets from the Early Cold War and Korea (Bloomington: Indiana University Press, 1998).

26 Li Dequan, "San nian lai Zhongguo renmin de weisheng shiye [The Chinese People's Health in the Past Three Years]," *Xinhua yuebao* [Xinhua Monthly], October 1951, 47.

27 Mao Zedong's inscription to the Second National Health Conference, December 1952.

28 Ka-che Yip, *Disease, Colonialism, and the State: Malaria in Modern East Asia* (Hong Kong: Hong Kong University Press, 2009), 8.

29 Chinese health posters: https://www.nlm.nih.gov/hmd/chineseposters/public.html.

30 Tuberculosis prevention posters: http://www.nlm.nih.gov/exhibition/chineseantitb/fourseries4.html.

31 Sigrid Schmalzer, *Red Revolution, Green Revolution: Scientific Farming in Socialist China* (Chicago: University of Chicago Press, 2016).

32 Liu Yingjie, *Zhongguo jiaoyu dashiji* [Major Events of Education in China] (Hangzhou: Zhejiang jiaoyu chubanshe, 1993), 1831; and Liao Qifa, *Dangdai Zhongguo saomang he nongcun chengren jiaoyu de huimo yu qianzhan* [Literacy and Adult Education in Contemporary Rural China] (Chongqing: Xinan shifan daxue chubanshe, 2002), 10–11.

33 Yu Bo and Xie Guodong, *Zhongguo saomang jiaoyu*, 6.

34 Liping Bu, "Anti-Malaria Campaigns and Socialist Reconstruction of China, 1950–1980" *East Asian History*, no. 39 (2014): 117–130. http://www.eastasianhistory.org/39/bu/index.html.

35 Longrui, "Xiangcun weisheng yuan de xunlian ji weishengshi de jianli [Training of Village Health Workers and the Establishment of Village Clinics]," *Huadong weisheng* [East China Health] 1, no. 2 (February 1951): 22.

36 Liping Bu and Elizabeth Fee, "Unite to Fight Malaria!" *American Journal of Public Health* 100, no. 4 (April 2010); and "Communicating with Pictures: The Vision of Chinese Anti-Malaria Posters," *American Journal of Public Health* 100, no. 3 (March 2010).

37 Nancy Tomes, "Moralizing the Microbe: The Germ Theory and the Moral Construction of Behavior in the Late Nineteenth Century Tuberculosis Movement," in *Morality and Health*, eds. Allan Brandt and Paul Rozin (London: Routledge, 1997); and Nancy Tomes, *The Gospel of Germs* (Cambridge, MA: Harvard University Press, 1998).

38 Tao-Tai Hsia, "Laws on Public Health," in *Medicine and Public Health in the People's Republic of China*, ed. Joseph R. Quinn (U.S. Department of Health, Education, and Welfare, Public Health Service, National Institutes of Health, 1973), 113–140. There was a timetable of target dates for the free medical service to be implemented in view of the uneven development and limited medical facilities in certain parts of the country, and other measures were also offered to cover medical expenses.

39 Tao-Tai Hsia, "Laws on Public Health," 128–130.

40 *Dangdai Zhongguo weisheng dashi ji* (1949-1990) [Major Events and Health Work in Contemporary China, 1949-1990] (Renmin weisheng chubanshe, 1993), 39.

41 Tu Changliang, "Feijiehe liaoyangyuan de guimo duomo da heshi [On the Proper Size of Sanatorium," *Fanglao tongxun* [*Anti-Tuberculosis Newsletter*], no. 4, 1956.

42 Liping Bu and Elizabeth Fee, "Get Well and Go Back to Work!" *American Journal of Public Health* 101, no. S1 (December, 2011): S165.

43 Chen Haifeng, *Zhongguo weisheng baojian shi*, 112.

44 Gao Xi, "Learning from the Soviet Union: Pavlovian Influence on Chinese Medicine, 1950s," in *Public Health and National Reconstruction in Post-War Asia:*

International Influences, Local Transformations, eds Liping Bu and Ka-che Yip (London: Routledge, 2015).

45 Kim Taylor, *Chinese Medicine in Early Communist China, 1945–1963* (London: Routledge, 2005); Kai Wai Fan, "Pavlovian Theory and the Scientification of Acupuncture in 1950s China," in *New Perspectives on the Research of Chinese Culture* (Springer, 2013).

46 China's anti-malaria campaign was not related to the WHO's worldwide malaria eradication program that was launched in 1955 during the Cold War. The WHO's program emphasized house spraying with residual insecticides, drug treatment, and surveillance, and successive steps of preparation, attack, consolidation and maintenance. Drug resistance, insecticide resistance, massive population movements, a lack of sustained funding, and inadequate community participation were cited as the difficulties in maintaining the long-term effort of eradication. The WHO abandoned the eradication campaign in 1968 and began a program of malaria control instead (Center for Disease Control and Prevention, Department of Health and Human Services, http://www.cdc.gov/Malaria, accessed August 15, 2019).

47 WHO news release, 30 June 2021, "From 30 million cases to zero: China is certified malaria-free by WHO." https://www.who.int/news/item/30-06-2021-from-30-million-cases-to-zero-china-is-certified-malaria-free-by-who. Accessed September 1, 2021.

48 Yue Qianhou and He Puyan, "Shanxi sheng Jishan xian nongcun gonggong weisheng shiye shuping (1949–1984)—Yi Taiyangcun (gongshe) wei zhongdian kaocha duixiang [Review of Rural Public Health of Jishan County, Shanxi Province, 1949–1984: A Case Study of Taiyangcun (Commune)]," *Dangdai Zhongguo shi yanjiu* 14, no. 5 (September 2007): 63.

49 Xia Xingzhen, "Nongcun hezuo yiliao zhidu de lishi kaocha [A Historical Study of Rural Medical Cooperatives]," *Dangdai Zhongguo shi yanjiu* 10, no. 5 (September 2003): 111.

50 Wang Sheng and Liu Yingqin, "Jitihua shiqi nongcun hezuo yiliao zhidu pingxi— Yi Hebei sheng Shenze xian wei ge an [An Analysis of Rural Medical Cooperative System during the Collectivization Era: A Case Study of Shenze County of Hebei Province," *Dangdai Zhongguo shi yanjiu* 16, no. 2 (March 2009): 26.

51 "Guanyu ba weisheng gongzuo zhongdian zhuanxiang nongcun de baogao [Report on Shifting the Emphasis of Health Work towards the Countryside," in *Nongcun weisheng wenjian huibian (1951–2000)*, 27.

52 Those who worked at collective industries and enterprises in cities and the countryside had collective healthcare rather than the state healthcare.

53 Yao Li, "'Ba yiliao weisheng gongzuo de zhongdian fang dao nongcun qu'—Mao Zedong's 'liu er liu' zhishi de lishi kaocha ["Put the Emphasis of Health Work in the Countryside"—A Historical Study of Mao Zedong's June 26 Instruction]," *Dangdai Zhongguo shi yanjiu* 14, no. 3 (May 2007): 99–104.

54 Zhu Chao and Zhang Weifeng, *Xin Zhongguo yixue jiaoyu shi* [History of Medical Education in the New China] (Beijing: Beijing yikedaxue and Zhongguo xiehe yikedaxue lianhe chubanshe, 1990), 111–140.

55 In the commune system, a commune usually had about 10 brigades and a brigade had about 10 production teams. Each production team had about 10–20 households.

56 Zhang Kaining, *Cong chijiao yisheng dao xiangcun yisheng* [From the Barefoot Doctor to the Village Doctor] (Yunnan renmin chubanshe, 2002), 17; and Li Decheng, "Xin Zhongguo qian sanshi nian jiceng weisheng renyuan peiyang moshi tanjiu [An Exploration of the Training Models for Basic-level Rural Health Workers in the First Thirty Years of the People's Republic of China]," *Dangdai Zhongguo shi yanjiu* 68, no. 2 (March 2009).

57 *Nongcun weisheng wenjian huibian* (1951-2000), 420.
58 Ibid., 533–534.
59 When the people's communes were dismantled in the 1980s, rural medical cooperatives and barefoot doctors stopped functioning.
60 Zhou Xun, *The People's Health: Health Intervention and Delivery in Mao's China, 1949–1983* (Montreal: McGill-Queen's University Press, 2020).
61 World Population Prospects, the 2008 Revision. United Nations, Department of Economic and Social Affairs (DESA), Population Division, New York. See www.unpopulation.org. China Profile, Analyses, Tables, Figures and Maps. http://www.china-profile.com/data/fig_WPP2008_L0_1.htm, accessed December 13, 2015.

2 Public Health as an Ideology for Socialistic Transformation of the Environment in North Korea, 1945–1961

The Case of Paragonimiasis Eradication

Junho Jung

Introduction

On November 13, 2017, major newspapers reported that dozens of round-worms were found in a North Korean soldier's ruptured small intestine during the treatment of a gunshot wound. The soldier had just defected through the Panmunjom Joint Security Area, and the political significance of the incident was not lost. Even a surgical scene to remove the roundworms from the rup-tured small intestine was shown on CNN in the United States.[1] This case was cited as an example of visualizing the reality of the collapsing North Korean health system, which has been deteriorating since the "Arduous March" in the 1990s.[2] It was reported that major epidemic diseases like cholera, malaria, typhoid fever, and tuberculosis have surged since the floods of 1995. With a limited supply of resources from the former Soviet Union, the North Korean government ordered to reduce material use in agriculture, by using less insec-ticides and returning back to night soil instead of chemical fertilizer. This change provided ideal conditions for the reemergence of parasitic diseases.[3]

According to the results of a survey conducted in North Korea by South Korean parasitologists in 2005, the overall infection rates among North Kore-ans still remained high. Stool examination of 236 North Koreans showed that the overall egg positivity rate was 57.6%, with roundworms 43.2%, and whip-worms 40.3%.[4] In 2004, a serological test for parasites of 270 North Koreans who arrived in South Korea showed a positive rate of 21.5%.[5] One notable point in this serological survey was that there was no paragonimiasis found, while other parasites prevailed.[6] It may be attributed to the small sample size, but considering that North Korea in the past was "one of the most prevalent places for paragonimiasis," it was unusual to find no paragonimiasis with a deteriorating public health system.[7]

Paragonimiasis in North Korea caused serious health problems in the 1950s. However, by the end of 1961, North Korea announced that paragoni-miasis had been eradicated.[8] The North Korean paragonimiasis eradication

DOI: 10.4324/9781003318163-3

project was a representative success story of early North Korean health care. The project was considered "an important struggle to assure the legitimacy of the party's preventive medical policy."[9] A series of executive orders were issued from 1955 onwards to "exterminate" paragonimiasis in North Korea.[10] The paragonimiasis eradication project was carried out by blocking all developmental stages of *Paragonimus* that existed in the ecosystem, and by using methods to treat and prevent each host, including humans. The theoretical basis of this project came from the Soviet experience of controlling dracunculiasis in the 1920s and 1930s, which was an ecological approach based on mass mobilization when it was difficult to use therapeutic agents or surgical interventions to eliminate parasitic diseases.[11] North Korean medical scientists, such as Ra Soon-young and Joo Sung-soon, adapted the Soviet theory to the North Korean situation, borrowed from China's experience of schistosomiasis eradication, and came up with a comprehensive system of a more ecological approach to tackle paragonimiasis and its eradication.

Most of the historical research on North Korean paragonimiasis eradication was done by North Korean scholars.[12] The paragonimiasis eradication project was such an important event in North Korea's public health history that it was treated as a significant separate item. Major secondary sources in North Korea since the 1970s, such as *The People's Father* (1975), *Public Health History in Korea* (1981), and *History of Korea* (1981), introduced paragonimiasis eradication as a major public health project in the 1950s.[13] In North Korean books on the history of medicine, paragonimiasis was the only one that was mentioned with a specific disease name. Just like the Chollima Movement, which emerged as a leading example of rapid economic development during the construction of North Korea's socialistic system, the paragonimiasis eradication project received significant attention as the success story of public health. Researchers in South Korea, however, refer to the paragonimiasis eradication project only fragmentarily in the process of examining North Korea's macro-medical system or in their epidemiological analysis of parasite infection rate surveys.[14]

Previous studies have focused on the political, economic, and ideological factors in the formation of the health system as socialist medical care in North Korea.[15] Few studies analyzed the nature of North Korea's health care by examining how North Koreans responded to individual diseases that hindered their socialistic nation building. The paragonimiasis eradication project was set in the 1950s when North Korea underwent transformation through ideological struggles in the society and collectively built a socialist state. The project mobilized people, health workers, and political leaders to collectively remodel the ecosystem in the process of eradicating the disease. This chapter examines the paragonimiasis eradication project during the socialist construction. It describes the social characteristics of North Korea and the ecological environment that caused health problems leading to the loss of labor. By examining the process of paragonimiasis eradication, this study shows how North Korea, which declared the completion of socialization of production in 1958, attempted socialist transformation of the entire ecosystem that formed the material basis of socialist life in addition to human transformation.[16] Furthermore, it examines how medical knowledge and practice were transferred and implemented in North Korea through the heterogeneous transnational network brought about by the Cold War. It shows how the connectivity of intellectual networks that were formed before the liberation from Japanese colonial rule created a new type of public health knowledge in North Korea, in spite of the separation of the two Koreas.

North Korea's Paragonimiasis Epidemic and the Crisis of Workforce

In the 1950s and 1960s, a variety of parasites were prevalent on the Korean Peninsula to the extent that it was called the "parasite kingdom."[17] In the public health effort to control diseases, North Korea focused on the epidemic of paragonimiasis rather than intestinal parasites such as roundworms and hookworms. The reason that North Korea concentrated on paragonimiasis was because of its unique symptoms that devastated the nation's labor force, particularly the male labor force. The most common symptom of paragonimiasis was coughing up blood (hemoptysis). Hemoptysis was often caused by particularly strenuous labor or exercise. When paragonimiasis reaches the final host, humans, it passes through the duodenum and penetrates into the abdominal cavity. In the abdominal cavity, paragonimiasis settles in the lungs where oxygen is high. However, as the route to the lungs is complicated, it often parasitizes the brain, the stomach, and the ovaries[18] In particular, cerebral paragonimiasis, in which *Paragonimus* disseminates to the brain, is fatal enough to cause 80% of deaths within 3 years.[19] Patients with cerebral conditions are considered "doomed to become disabled and paralyzed.[20] Cerebral paragonimiasis accounts for 42% of all infections.[21] One of the main characteristics of paragonimiasis is its interference in the workforce by consuming labor with hemoptysis or severe neurological symptoms. Infected men showed the epidemiologic characteristics that caused depletion of labor in North Korea when the country was pushing for fast economic development.

Paragonimus infects humans through two intermediate hosts, the first being freshwater snails and the second being crabs and crayfish. Although it was most commonly transmitted to humans when people ingested larvae-infected crabs and crayfish without proper cooking, studies in North Korea found that people became infected by drinking the water that was contaminated with larvae.[22] The habits of eating marinated crabs or crushed crayfish were cited as major factors for infection and prevalence of paragonimiasis in the Korean Peninsula.[23] In the past, when children contracted measles or had a nosebleed, the custom was to feed them crushed raw crayfish as a cure.[24] Due to these folk remedies, the prevalence of paragonimiasis often reached its peak following the year of a measles epidemic.[25] Boys were more likely to engage in risky behaviors such as "swimming in rivers, especially in the summer," or "eating incompletely roasted crayfish" when they were young. "Marinated crabs were a rare delicacy" and were given preferentially to adult males as a treat.[26] Due to these traditional cultural customs, the infection rate of paragonimiasis was higher among men than among women. The infection rate was also highest among men of 13 to 15 years old and after the age of 20.[27]

Paragonimiasis was particularly prevalent in the northern part of Korea. According to the epidemiologic surveys of paragonimiasis conducted by the Japanese colonial government in the 1920s, the infection rate was relatively low in the southern part of the Korean Peninsula, with Gyeonggi having 10.4%; Gyeongbuk, 6.2%; and Jeonnam, 4.6%.[28] The infection rate in the northern part, however, was as high as 23.1% in Hwanghae and 18.7% in Pyeongnam. A survey on the prevalence of paragonimiasis conducted in North Korea in 1954 found that paragonimiasis was endemic across the whole nation.[29] In the Sinheung district of South Pyongan Province, 63.2% of the residents were infected, and in the Sinsang district of South Hamgyong Province, 76.4% of the subjects were tested positive for paragonimiasis.[30]

In the mid-1950s, when North Korea was undergoing postwar recovery and fast economic development, it decided to eradicate paragonimiasis because it so crippled people that they "cannot even farm."[31] Treating paragonimiasis patients became "an important means of actively mobilizing the masses to realize the Party's health policy by restoring their ability to work."[32] Kim Il-sung directly instructed people that the "struggle for paragonimiasis eradication should be powerfully initiated across the nation and among the people."[33] During the Chollima Movement for national recovery, it was an important task to "prevent" all diseases, including infectious diseases, and to reduce "the temporary loss of workers' ability to work."[34] To achieve the goals, all health workers directed their attention to paragonimiasis eradication. They led this fight against parasites "at a time when all the workers are rushing toward the hill of socialism with the momentum of Chollima."[35]

Searching for the Methods of Eradication: "Devastation" Approach

Ra Soon-young (1919–2005) was one of the few parasitologists in Korea who, shortly after the Korean War broke out, moved to North Korea. There, he served as head of the Department of Parasitology at Pyongyang Medical University and the director of the Parasitology Research Office of the Ministry of Health. He led the field of parasitology in North Korea, borrowed the experience and theories of Soviet and Chinese parasite eradication, and applied them to paragonimiasis control in North Korea. In particular, he synthesized Soviet theoretical concepts and experience with the scientific knowledge he had learned from Japan when he was a student.

Ra graduated from the Faculty of Medicine at Keijo Imperial University (京城帝國大學) in 1943. The Department of Parasitology in Keijo University was led by Kobayashi Harujiro (小林晴治郎), who was the first to have identified freshwater carps as the intermediate hosts of paragonimiasis in 1916.[36] With the influence of Kobayashi, parasitologists in Korea during the colonial period actively participated in paragonimiasis research.[37] Identification of the intermediate hosts led to the prevention effort of catching snails, banning eating raw freshwater fish, and administering experimental emetin drugs.[38] Korea was at the forefront of paragonimiasis knowledge production.

Ra Soon-young published a textbook on paragonimiasis in 1955 that covered the basic morphology and physiology of the parasite and treatment and prevention based on up-to-date research from Japan, the Soviet Union, China, and the United States.[39] On the epidemiological history in Korean Peninsula and the life cycle of *Paragonimus westermani*, Ra cited works by Japanese parasitologists during the colonial period, but he harshly criticized that much of the epidemiological data collected by the colonial government were "irresponsible and incorrect" as they were based on sputum tests only.[40] In the chapters on chemotherapy and prevention, he focused on works from China and the Soviet Union. As China actively engaged in research and control activities of epidemic diseases in the early 1950s, cutting-edge knowledge on chemotherapy and clinical symptoms was provided by Chinese scholars, notably Zhong Huilan (钟惠澜).[41] It included diagnosis through antigenic test and combination therapy of emetin and other drugs.[42] Although earlier works from Japanese scholars during the colonial period provided primary knowledge regarding the basic biology of the parasite, limited progress was made in interventions. Japanese health officials tried emetin treatment in late 1920s' Korea, but this experiment resulted in six deaths from the adverse reaction of chemotherapy, and so they later faced public resistance to the treatment.[43] The frontline of knowledge production regarding parasitology shifted from Japan to China when China sought active control of parasitic diseases.

Since 1945, North Korea's healthcare was greatly influenced by medical support from the Soviet Union, China, and socialist countries of Eastern Europe. The Eastern Bloc medical teams not only procured equipment and materials but also took charge of educating North Korean medical personnel in educational and intellectual exchanges. After 1951, especially with the claims of American use of biological weapons in the Korean War, experts in infectious disease and hygiene were dispatched to North Korea from the Soviet Union more frequently. This involved Polina Andreevna Petrishcheva, a member of the Parasitology Department of the Academy of Medicine and an expert in vector control in the Soviet Union.[44] Lenke Horvath, a neurosurgeon from Romania, also took great interest in cerebral paragonimiasis. They conducted research with North Korean doctors on surgical treatment and control measures since 1952.[45]

The Soviet expertise on parasitological disease control provided theoretical ground for Ra, who was aware of the limitations of chemotherapy for postwar reconstruction. Chemotherapy, with emetin, caused severe side effects and required trained medical personnel for administering the treatment. At the suggestion of Soviet scholars, Ra, instead, focused on the interruption of the parasite's life cycle in the ecosystem as the feasible approach to tackle paragonimiasis. In Ra's view, the previous model of interventions taken by Japan relied on passive case finding and post-exposure treatment, whereas the Soviet model took more active measures to interrupt the contact between humans and parasites in the first place. In the latter half of his book, Ra described preventive measures taken by the Soviets during the first half of the 20th century in great detail, focusing on the concept of "Devastation (девастачия)" and "Prophylaxis (профилактика)." The method was originally proposed by the Soviet parasitologist, Konstantin Ivanovich Skrjabin, based on his observation of the ecology of various parasites in a geographical survey spanning across the Soviet Union.[46] Thereafter, extensive ecological knowledge of parasites became the basis for the ecological approach in Soviet parasite control.[47]

In the Soviet experience, Bukhara in Uzbekistan was one of the major endemic areas of dracunculiasis. In Bukhara, when the dracunculiasis eradication project began in 1923, the prevalence rate was 20% of the population with over 10,000 cases reported.[48] Based on the data collected from Bukhara, Skrjabin proposed the theory of deworming (дегельминтизации) in 1925.[49] This theory, which was the prototype of Devastation, had the key concept of "environment improvement through systematic therapeutic intervention." The concept was to reduce the number of parasites in the environment by reducing egg contamination in the ecosystem and the preventive measures of thoroughly blocking the cause of contamination, that is, parasitic eggs.

The dracunculiasis eradication project, which implemented the "deworming" approach, emphasized ecological intervention such as blocking the contact between people and crustacean vectors through hydraulic engineering modification of wells and ponds. The education of residents was carried out to raise their intensive awareness, and anyone confirmed to be infected was completely banned from going to the well until treatment was complete.[50] More extreme measures like pouring oil into contaminated wells to make them completely unusable were carried out as well. Water use was only allowed in areas that were confirmed to have been completely treated by a locally appointed "water officer."[51] There was even extensive culling of dogs, as they were a major link to the transmission. In 1931, 9 years after the eradication program that attacked all stages of parasitic transmission, only one case of infection was reported.[52]

Skrjabin's deworming concept was further refined through the experience of dracunculiasis eradication across the Soviet Union in the 1920s and 1930s.[53] Based on these experiences, the concept of "Devastation," which meant the management of all stages of parasite development, was presented, at the General Assembly of the Soviet Academy of Sciences in October 1944.[54] The 1947 publication, "Devastation in the Fight against Nematodes and Other Human and Animal Diseases," extended the concept to the fight against protozoan and bacterial diseases.[55]

Devastation was "active and aggressive preventive methods to attack and eradicate parasites by using all possible methods for all stages of the life cycle of the parasite, from eggs to larva to adult development in entirety."[56] By comparison, "prophylaxis" refers to "a passive and defensive preventive method that does not attack the pathogen itself, but protects the human and animal host organism from the invasion of parasites."[57] In other words, Devastation was a concept that emphasized the need to intervene in the overall external ecosystem that causes parasite infection, beyond the passive level of prevention such as the treatment of patients and the protection of noninfected people. In essence, the Devastation project in the USSR was extensive state intervention and mass mobilization based on scientific research, by intensively utilizing all the capabilities of community health and medical resources surrounding the infection route.

Ra criticized the previous "preventive medicine point of view," which emphasized the individualistic treatment of the disease in paragonimiasis eradication.[58] The individualized treatment did not suppress the density of the parasite in the ecosystem, and continuous reexposure and reinfection wasted "valuable drugs."[59] Previous public health measures narrowly focused on the treatment of the disease rather than holistic interventions to improve health in general.[60] Insufficient results from the past were due to passively providing treatments with no systematic connection of the concept of prophylaxis and devastation in wider ecology. Ra argued that a comprehensive consideration of patients and carriers was needed in an eradiation system that would simultaneously protect the healthy people and treat the patients as well as tackling the pathogens in the external environment.[61] In addition, he pointed out that a policy of restricting major protein sources such as crab and crayfish should be considered in order to change people's disease perception and the eating habits of people in mountainous regions who "believe that paragonimiasis is a fatal disease that comes from the local waters and soils."[62] In order to annihilate the intermediate hosts in a Devastation manner, it was necessary to understand the regional life cycle and the epidemic characteristics of paragonimiasis and residents so as to apply the optimal fighting method.[63]

While the theoretical background of the anti-paragonimiasis work was adopted from the Soviets, details of the actual implementation knowledge were in line with Chinese anti-schistosomiasis work. Schistosomiasis became the focus of public health work in China in 1950. With support from the Soviets, China dedicated much of the effort to research and surveys in the early phase from 1950 to 1955. The implantation of the schistosomiasis control program was placed in junction with the Patriotic Public Health Program, which allowed the Chinese government to build a network of designated epidemic disease prevention stations for the campaign.[64]

As the largest economic aid provider, along with the Soviets, China provided much of the technical assistance to North Korea during the 1950s.[65] Although details of the support have yet to be elucidated with more archival materials, Ra's book published in 1955 shows the influence of the Chinese experience: placing a network of centers for parasitic diseases control in endemic localities, grassroots mobilization through political party, and an extensive survey on the prevalence of the disease.

From Theory to Practice: Implementation of Paragonimiasis Prevention and Treatment, 1955–1958

Although Ra had provided the necessary theoretical framework for paragonimiasis control, it needed to be proven in the field to demonstrate that it was applicable in North Korean settings. Joo Sung-soon, a pathologist, was the first to use the Devastation method in the real world. Joo also was in a unique position to integrate knowledge from neighboring countries. Graduated from Keijo College of Medicine (京城醫學專門學校) in 1940, he worked in China until Korea's liberation from Japanese colonial rule in 1945. He moved to North Korea during the Korean War and became a professor at Hamheung Medical School in 1954.[66] There, he was able to combine the "experiences from China's schistosomiasis eradication plan" with the "Skrjabin's Devastation methods from the Soviets" for a comprehensive program of total elimination of paragonimiasis in the Hamkyung province.[67] Since 1949, China had implemented a nationwide schistosomiasis control program that sought to mobilize people at the grassroots level to catch snails, the intermediate host.[68]

In 1954, Joo established a temporary prevention center for paragonimiasis in selected villages for a pilot program, and conducted extensive epidemiological surveys on the climate, soil, fauna and flora, local customs, working conditions, water supply, toilets, residential areas, and diet, among other epidemiologically significant factors.[69] Similar to what had been done in Bukhara, the center did water-source management, collection and control of the intermediate hosts, and culling of the animal reservoir of the disease, such as dogs. Health workers from the prevention center did door-to-door visits in the village for advocacy, testing, and case history taking. Within 2 years of the pilot program, they observed a significant reduction in the infection rate with aggressive Devastation intervention. Some of the key lessons were the necessity of identifying epidemiological characteristics in the local region, training mid-level health workers, conducting ecological interventions such as removing snails, using visual materials for educational advocacy, and involving key political partners in the region.

One of the key developments was the advancement in diagnostic techniques that made mass screening possible. Previously, sputum testing was mainly used as a method for diagnosing paragonimiasis. The sputum test was the most accurate method for diagnosing currently infected patients because it directly detected eggs. However, there were a few limitations of the method.[70] During the early stage of infection, eggs were not detected in sputum. In the case of children, they had difficulty in collecting sputum. Also, the process of collecting sputum from each examinee and sending it to a laboratory for diagnosis under a microscope required trained personnel. However, the newly developed intradermal antigen-reaction method was performed by extracting antigens from the *Paragonimus westermani*, diluting them in saline, and then examining the skin reactions after intradermal injection. With the antigen-test method, it was possible to check the test results in 15 minutes, and it did not require professional personnel such as microscopists, hence allowing mass examination of large numbers of people within a short time.[71] However, due to the nature of the immune-response test, it was difficult to discern the current infection from the past infection. Nevertheless, technological advances such as the intradermal antigen test provided an important basis for identifying major epidemic areas and confirming their epidemiologic characteristics. Along with the epidemiologic survey of humans, an investigation was also carried out to specifically identify the types and density of intermediate hosts by distinguishing them from headwaters and tributaries.[72] The identification of regional epidemiologic characteristics of paragonimiasis through mass examination was the first step in carrying out the "Devastation-style struggle principle."[73]

As the pilot program on paragonimiasis control made significant progress, North Korean leaders became confident and adopted Cabinet Order No. 9 on February 9, 1955, titled "On Organization and Implementation of Paragonimiasis Prevention and Treatment Measures."[74] The Order instructed people to bury crabs and crayfish in paragonimiasis endemic areas and banned raw consumption of them.[75] Although the North Korean government at that time claimed that the paragonimiasis eradication project was "organized in close connection with the pilot project and practical countermeasures," national implementation of the "countermeasures" used in the pilot project was hindered by a number of difficulties.[76]

The Devastation project provided protection for noninfected people through the improvement of the local living environment, the complete eradication of the intermediate host through ecosystem modification, and the active treatment of the currently infected patients simultaneously. According to the investigation, there were five routes through which eggs excreted from patients contaminated the external environment: first, when sputum was spit directly into a creek; second, when sputum spit on the road went into a stream with rainwater; third, washing containers that were contaminated with sputum; fourth, when feces containing the eggs went into the water; and, fifth, feces excreted along the stream that was washed in.[77] Paragonimiasis was a disease that could be sufficiently prevented if only the known transmission routes of eggs were blocked, but health workers and facilities capable of carrying out these activities were still insufficient in rural areas. Unlike intestinal parasites such as roundworms that were easily visible, paragonimiasis, which live in the lungs, were not easily excreted from the body. They had a complicated life cycle in humans via the infection route of crabs and crayfish. It made them less visible to human eyes and difficult to attribute the disease risk to specific parasites.

For patient treatment, "precious drugs that were not yet produced in Korea had to be purchased with valuable foreign currency."[78] Moreover, they showed limited effectiveness despite the high price.[79] With no alternative available, emetin-injection therapy remained the choice of treatment for paragonimiasis, even though it was highly toxic and required a long treatment period. The emetin regime required 15 to 20 days of administration, a rest for about 20 days, and started again when the cumulative toxicity was relieved, and this cycle had to be performed up to five times. Because of the high toxicity, it was necessary to carefully adjust the dose according to the body weight, with necessary medical professional oversight. In 1955, when the paragonimiasis eradication project began, North Korea was in a three-year period of economic recovery and focusing on securing a number of medical facilities and manpower. With a severe shortage of medical resources, wide application of emetin was unrealistic.[80] It was after 1956 when primary clinics were established at agricultural cooperatives and villages that the necessary oversight of medical professionals became possible at the local level.

As a way to overcome the limitations of medical resources, North Korea prioritized mobilizing the public to remove the intermediate hosts, such as crayfish, crabs, and snails.[81] Although it was possible to prevent further contamination by improving the local sanitation environment, it was difficult to contain the large numbers of larvae already present in the intermediate hosts of local ecosystems. Therefore, the Soviet Devastation-style method was proposed that included the collection of hosts through mass mobilization, the hydraulic engineering of remodeling waterways of rivers, the chemical method of using molluscicide, and the biological method of controlling snails by livestock (such as ducks) feeding on the snails but were not infected by paragonimiasis.

In particular, snail collection was intensively performed because larvae could rapidly proliferate in the snail by asexual reproduction, which had a decisive effect on the infection rate of the second intermediate hosts and humans.[82] Also, snails were relatively easy to collect as they mostly lived in rivers, compared to crayfish and crabs, which were mobile and distributed in the mountain regions.[83]

Collecting snails required a significant workforce with mobilization. Women and students were the primary targets of mobilization because they were considered a "reserve workforce." Reduction in aid from the Soviets since 1956 shifted North Korea's economic plan to "mobilization of internal reserves" to utilize domestic resources rather than relying on external support.[84] Through schools and women's groups, health workers provided visual educational materials about actual parasite specimens.[85] They brought microscopes to show the public living juvenile parasites in contaminated water and dissected infected intermediate hosts.[86] People in endemic regions used to say "water is too bad to live with," and "this local disease is incurable." They took it as if they were destined to be paralyzed by the disease simply because they lived in the area.[87] Now, with visual material teaching them about the inconspicuous parasites, people began to change their perception of paragonimiasis from an unavoidable natural phenomenon to a disease that could be treated.[88]

Visualization of the parasite "sensitized students" to deliver the message to their parents about the importance of eradicating the disease.[89] During the participation in collecting snails and other mobilization programs, health workers often promoted competitions between classes or groups with prizes.[90] Similar approaches were used by local political leaders as well. They used to be hesitant about mass mobilization when it seemed "impossible to catch all the snails."[91] With the advancement in diagnosis, health workers were able to identify local leaders who were infected with paragonimiasis and targeted those leaders with visual education materials. When the infected leaders changed their views and attitude after learning the scientific information about paragonimiasis, they became active in mobilizing local cooperatives, unions, and schools.

Medical school students and faculties were actively mobilized to fight the disease. Medical professionals who resisted the menial jobs of collecting snails were criticized as "old intelligentsia" not suitable for the socialist nation. Articles in *Inmin pogŏn* (People's Public Health) repeatedly portrayed heroic efforts of medical students getting involved in public health activities with villagers. The old intelligentsia who thought it was not the "doctor's job" to collect snails were reeducated with experience in rural areas. In other words, the development and success of the paragonimiasis eradication project in the 1950s also demonstrated the party's use of the public health campaign, in the ideological struggle, to convert the intelligentsia into socialistic workers to serve the party and the people.

In rural areas of North Korea where paragonimiasis was prevalent, cooperative organizations were still in the formative stage in 1955 and were not fully incorporated into the national administrative system. Therefore, health workers faced difficulties in conducting active mass mobilization on large-scale interventions.[92] This was partly due to the lack of political will of local party leaders and partly due to the public's lack of understanding of diseases. In 1956, North Korea completed the three-year plan of economic recovery, and in 1957, when the first five-year plan began, medical facilities and manpower significantly surpassed pre-war levels. The Cabinet Order of August 1956, "On the Improvement and Strengthening of People's Health Work," revealed that compared to 1945, the number of hospital beds increased 14.4 times and the number of treatment and prevention institutions increased 27.6 times. The same order attributed the lack of satisfactory results in the health sector to "the health administration [that] guided people in a narrow and manual way with only the power of health workers, instead of actively bringing the masses into the health work through extensive mass political mobilization."[93] The order instructed to make "the people fully realize that the people's health project is their own business and they should actively participate in the project." This means that the government now demanded active mass mobilization to carry out large-scale Devastation-style projects that could not be done by health workers alone. In addition, the organization of agricultural cooperatives was promoted rapidly in early 1956. The agricultural cooperative ratio, which remained at 49% in December 1955, surged to 65.6% in February 1956 and 80.9% in December, while agricultural productivity rapidly surpassed pre-war levels.[94] In 1957, 30 paragonimiasis prevention centers were also established in major epidemic areas; and hence, the foundation for paragonimiasis eradication project was laid in rural areas.[95]

With the rapid socialist changes in rural North Korea that occurred in 1956 and the expansion of medical facilities, medical technology also advanced significantly. Technological development in the field of parasitology at Hamhung Medical School and Hygiene Research Institute once again provided the leadership for paragonimiasis eradication to be actively carried out across North Korea. The "Emethine-Chloroquine Combination Therapy" and "Vaccine-Emethine-Chloroquine Combination Therapy" were created as methods to reduce the adverse reaction of emetine and shorten the treatment period.[96] According to the survey conducted in Yodok in 1956, the relapse rate among those using the newly introduced combination therapy dropped to 16%, which was much lower than that of the existing emetine monotherapy of 35% to 40%.[97] Studies on the natural course of paragonimiasis from 1954 to 1957 showed optimistic results that parasites could actually be eradicated within a shorter period. They showed that the annual spontaneous cure rate of paragonimiasis was 26.9%, and it was hypothesized that if there was no reinfection for 4 years, most people would spontaneously heal and the infection route would be naturally blocked.[98] The emergence of more efficient treatment and the expansion of health facilities made it possible to treat existing patients, and the formation of rural cooperatives laid the foundation for mass mobilization to eradicate intermediate hosts and improve the local environment.

Sanitation Work as an All-People's Movement, 1958–1961

On May 4, 1958, Kim Il-sung emphasized, at the Standing Committee of the Workers' Party of Korea, that "in the provinces with many paragonimiasis cases such as North and South Hwanghae, the deputy ministers should directly take responsibility and guide this project."[99] On May 19, 1958, the Cabinet issued Order No. 52, "On Organizational Development of Sanitation Work as an All-People's Movement."[100] The government decided to eradicate paragonimiasis within 3 years. The Order directed that provincial People's Committees and the Ministries of Home Affairs, Culture, Chemical Industry, Defense and Commerce cooperate with the health sector to carry out their respective roles in the paragonimiasis eradication movement. Leaders of People's Committees of paragonimiasis-infected regions instructed people to construct new wells and latrines and clean up rivers to eradicate intermediate hosts in a mass movement. Agricultural cooperatives were to play a key role in strengthening the paragonimiasis control effort. Scattered households that were difficult to renovate, educate, or treat at the local level were to be relocated into collective villages and incorporated into the eradication program.

In August 1958, when all the individual farmers were integrated into agricultural cooperatives and the conversion to socialist mode of production was completed in rural areas, mass mobilization in rural areas became more intensive.[101] The Ministries of Defense, Home Affairs, Education, and Culture were given the authority to mobilize military units, students, and all faculty and students at medical colleges. Hence, the groundwork for mobilization was carried out not only among rural residents but also among all the different groups of the workforce. The Ministry of Chemical Industry was in charge of the production of emetine, and the Ministry of Commerce ordered the import of emetine raw materials and sent to paragonimiasis endemic areas supplies of anthracite coal for boiling water.[102]

Paragonimiasis prevention centers were established to take charge of the eradication project so that "Devastation" methods could be implemented comprehensively in rural areas.[103] Starting with 30 centers in 1957, the number increased to 332 in 1958 and 698 in 1959 in different locations.[104] The use of prevention centers to launch Devastation method was also influenced by the Soviet experience of malaria eradication in the early 1950s when there was a surge of malaria following World War II. In the malaria-eradication project, the Soviets used a "dispensarization" control method via a network of malaria-prevention stations as well as the management of mosquito larvae through extensive hydraulic modification. The method was to use the dense network of prevention centers to conduct mass checkups and actively monitor and treat the infected persons with follow-up treatment.[105]

The economic, scientific, and technical support of China was crucial in this period. Beginning in late 1957, diplomatic relations between North Korea and China gradually improved. In junction with the Chollima Movement and the Great Leap Forward in 1958, China greatly increased its aid to North Korea from February 1958. Also in October, they signed an agreement to establish the science and technology commission.[106] The economic and scientific aid from China allowed a rapid implementation of the nationwide anti-paragonimiasis during this crucial period.

Based on epidemiological surveys, treatment was to be performed compulsorily for all patients at regular intervals, rather than different strategies for individual patients, and for all infected residents of the epidemic area.[107] To recruit specialists to work in the newly established prevention centers, the Cabinet issued Order No. 69 on July 21, 1958, "On the Guarantee to Train Specialists in the Prevention and Treatment of Paragonimiasis and Secondary Health Workers."[108] The government established a training center dedicated for the paragonimiasis prevention and treatment specialists from secondary school graduates and planned to train 1,000 auxiliary physicians annually.[109] After completing 150 hours of classes in Pyongyang, including professional knowledge on paragonimiasis, sanitation, parasitology, epidemiology, and clinical studies, nurses were dispatched to endemic areas to teach rural hygiene culture.[110] Training centers for paramedics were also set up in central hospitals

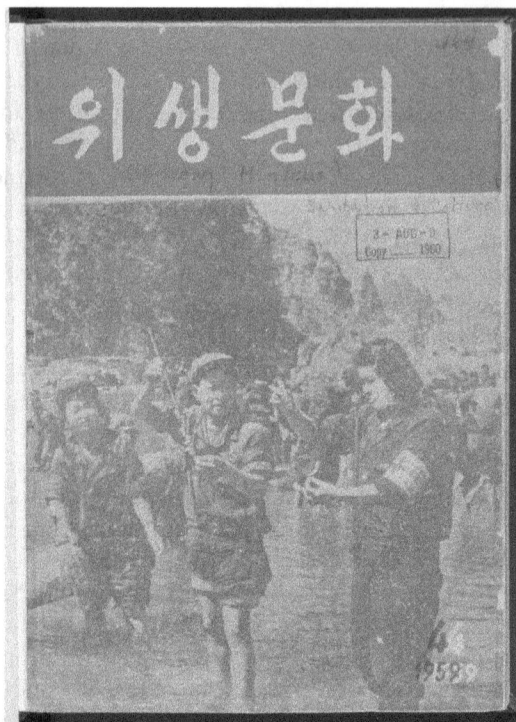

Figure 2.1 Students gathered along the river with local health workers to catch
        crayfish.

Source: Wisaeng munhwa, April 1959, Cover page.

in each province, and reeducation for secondary health workers have been
conducted since 1959 (Figure 2.1).[111]

As the parasite eradication was organized around the prevention centers
and human resources were secured, the paragonimiasis eradication project
began to "develop as a mass movement" in 1959.[112] Central to the project was
snail collection, which used a mechanical method to "scrape up the riverbed to
collect snails."[113] Since crayfish and crabs only came out at night, people had
to use torches to catch them.[114] In the Kaesong district, 22.3 tons of snails and
290 kilograms of crayfish were caught.[115]

At the National Health Workers' Meeting in 1959, the Central Committee
of the Workers' Party of Korea instructed to "actively introduce advanced
medical technology" and "systematize and disseminate widely all the achievements and experiences already achieved in our country."[116] As inter-ministerial
cooperation was required, most of the local labor force, including "all scouts,
youth groups, military personnel, and civil servants" were mobilized to collect
intermediate hosts.[117] By 1959, the Chollima Movement was well established
in the health sector, demanding old intelligentsia doctors to put prevention

above treatment, reach out to patients rather than sitting in the hospital, and uphold socialist ideology over technical skills.[118] Doctors were criticized for focusing on research that was too isolated from the real world or narrowly focused on medical technology over socialistic ideology. Devastation for paragonimiasis was an ideal means for the state to prove that the old intelligentsia doctors had become socialist workers, going into the field for preventive intervention while learning from people's experience on the grassroots level.[119] Hamheung Medical School students went to rural areas of Jagang Province to conduct surveys and eradicate intermediate hosts. Over 2 days in Jagang Province, 500 medical school students and staff caught 331,000 snails and 35,000 crayfish.[120] In Changseong-gun, 37 tons of intermediate hosts were caught over 4 months, by 500 students from the county.[121] In the same location, 10,000 people per year applied hydraulic engineering methods such as river remodeling to eradicating a total of 51 tons of intermediate hosts, including 6.6 tons of snails.

In addition to the mass mobilization of people, the natural eco-biological approach of using ducks to feed on snail vectors of paragonimiasis was another actively recommended method. This methods was first experimented in the Soviet Union in 1946 to target the type of snails transmitting flukes to cows.[122] While there was a risk that major livestock such as pigs could become infected with paragonimiasis and cause reinfection in humans, ducks were resistant to infection, and therefore the method could proceed "with the enforcement of our party's decision to develop the livestock industry."[123] Moreover, people's eating habits of crabs and crayfish could be effectively changed by actively encouraging the breeding of ducks to diversify protein sources within the region.[124] There were challenges, however, because the main food for ducks was not snails or crayfish. North Koreans solved the problems by modifying the diet of ducks to favor the intermediate hosts such as snails and crayfish.[125]

At first, I gave the ducks crushed snails and crayfish, but they didn't eat them at all. As the next method, the ducks were locked in a barn and only fed with snails and crayfish, so they started eating. After that, only the big ones were crushed, and the smaller ones were just given to them. They ate them all. After a few days, the ducks became accustomed to eating snails and crayfish. From then on, in the morning, flocks of ducks were driven to the river or stream. Ducks ate snails and crayfish in rivers and streams all day long.[126]

Ducks whose diet had been modified in this way were released into rivers or streams so that they would eat snails and crayfish to eradicate the intermediate hosts.[127] In the meantime, the production of ducks as livestock increased when snails and crayfish were collected to feed ducks during river cleaning. As more ducks were raised for the eradication of intermediate hosts, some unintended effects also happened. Parasitic trematode in ducks (*Echinostoma revolutum*) caused "parasitic castration" in snails. This trematode, which did not infect humans and only infected snails, destroyed the reproductive organs of the infected snails and sterilized them. Health workers released 60 trematode-infected ducks in every 10-kilometer section of the river, which led to the eradication of snails within 2 years.[128]

While the treatment of infected patients centered on the prevention center network and the "extermination attack" on intermediate hosts through mass mobilization, the final link of the Devastation project was environmental improvement and advocacy to prevent reinfection.[129] Kim Il-sung pointed out that "as is the case with all diseases, in the case of paragonimiasis, a long-standing endemic disease, good hygiene enlightenment and sanitation reform is a very important issue in eradicating this disease."[130] In the 1958 government directive, "On the Organization of Sanitation Work as an All-People's Movement," health workers were urged to

> provide extensive explanation and education about the route of infection and the preventive measures to the residents of areas where paragonimiasis was endemic, and at the same time carry out the construction and renovation of wells and toilets and the cleanup of rivers.[131]

Sanitary reforms such as the establishment of wells and toilets were deployed as part of the hygiene-culture project implemented in 1958, and the advocacy for eradication of paragonimiasis was also fully initiated.[132] Wherever there was a landline, the knowledge of paragonimiasis was disseminated through broadcast. In South Pyongan Province, sputum bins were built around all roads in the county as well as at homes to prevent infection through sputum from patients. Residents greeted each other in the morning saying, "Are you drinking boiled water?" and even when they went to work, they were seen carrying a bucket of boiled water.[133]

People became active participants in hygiene reform and in the intermediate collection of hosts. They said that eradication of paragonimiasis was "a thing that could only happen under the socialist system."[134] The paragonimiasis eradication project, through successful public mobilization, was praised for "a wide-ranging installation of paragonimiasis prevention centers, systematic free treatment for patients, a wide range of preventive measures, and a mass intermediate host eradication campaign."[135] It was reported that 74% of patients were cured and the intermediate hosts were basically eradicated across the nation.[136] As a result of those projects, it was declared that paragonimiasis was completely eradicated in all regions of North Korea at the end of 1961.[137] In the 1960s, the Devastation method of paragonimiasis eradication was applied to the effort to "completely eradicate intestinal parasites and harmful insects within the foreseeable future."[138] After the paragonimiasis eradication, the prevention centers were converted into clinics in rural areas, resulting in the expansion of public health facilities to a grassroots administrative level.[139]

Another unexpected outcome of paragonimiasis eradication was the impact on the field of parasitology in the Soviet Union. Although the Soviets had significantly advanced knowledge and experiences in parasitology, actual cases were rarely seen in hospital settings, leaving the younger generation of doctors inexperienced. During their time in North Korea, Soviet parasitologists gained access to rich research materials, revitalizing the field of tropical medicine.[140] In the case of Lenke Horvath from Romania, who helped found the field of neurosurgery in North Korea, she obtained significant expertise in experimental surgery by exploring the treatment of cerebral paragonimiasis when she was in North Korea.[141] The successful implementation of tackling infectious disease from theory to practice in North Korea had lasting impact within and across national borders.

Conclusion

This case study of paragonimiasis eradication demonstrates that disease control was one of the important facets of North Korea's public health improvement during the early socialist construction period. It shows North Korea's adaptation of the Soviet concept of Devastation theory and China's experience of schistosomiasis eradication to its own particular conditions, with the foundation of basic knowledge established by Japanese scholars during the colonial period. In the process of knowledge adaption and appropriation, North Korea's own research capabilities of medical scientists, such as Ra Soon-Young and Joo Sung-soon, were able to use localized epidemiological and biological surveys of paragonimiasis to create effective prevention and treatment measures for the eradication project. As most of the parasite experts on the Korean Peninsula moved to North Korea after the Korean War, North Korea was able to muster its health professional resources to carry out nationwide parasite control activities in the 1950s, earlier than South Korea but during the same period in China. The difference between the two Koreas mirrored the difference in the newly formed intellectual networks between the East and West in the Cold War geopolitics.

The theory of Devastation was reflected in the policy, applied to the field, and spread rapidly to health workers through education about prevention and treatment at training centers and medical schools. The characteristics of health and medical personnel in the paragonimiasis eradication also showed the field-oriented nature that was emphasized in North Korea during the Chollima Movement.[142] The health workers channeled the party's policy that required the research to be "closer to the real life of the people"[143] by conducting research and treatment in the field, and away from the passivity of working "only in university lectures, research institutes, or scientific academies."[144] After the transformation to the socialist mode of production was completed in 1958, the scope of socialist transformation was going beyond the social structures and people's views. It aimed at remodeling the entire ecosystem that formed the material basis of socialist life. As in the case of the ducks that were trained to eat the intermediate hosts of crabs and crayfish, which were not their originally preferred diet, the scope of environmental reformation broadened from people to other ecological beings.

This emphasis on ecological intervention, which set the North Korean parasite control program apart from the Chinese counterpart, was the by-product of political conflict. In August 1956, Kim Il-sung purged many of his political opponents and competitors in the party, known as the August Incidents. These factions had political ties with China and the Soviet Union. As economic dependency of the two big countries grew, the two factions started to threaten the sole leadership of Kim. After the purge Kim emphasized the independence of the nation, leading to the slogan of *juche*, self-reliance.[145] While Ra's writing in 1955 referenced much of the evidence to Chinese and Soviet scholars, articles on paragonimiasis in *Inmin pogŏn* after 1956 showed no mention of external support. The ecological elements of the North Korean paragonimiasis program were efforts to differentiate their program from the Chinese program of schistosomiasis while, at the same time, present it as the pinnacle of North Korean ingenuity, or *juche*, in public health.

Notes

1 Paula Newton and Taehoon Lee. "North Korean Soldier: Surgeon Says the Defector 'Was like a Broken Jar.'" *CNN*, December 5, 2017.
2 The "Arduous March" was the period between 1996 and 2000, when North Korea suffered severe economic hardship and famine. The combination of political instability after the death of Kim Il-sung and the severe famine following a series of draughts and flooding in 1994 exacerbated North Korea with further isolation from the rest of the world after the collapse of the Soviet Union. It was estimated that approximately 500,000 to 600,000 people died of hunger from 1993 to 2000, and life expectancy fell by 7 years. Daniel Goodkind, Loraine West and Peter Johnson, "A reassessment of mortality in North Korea, 1993–2008" (Paper presented at the Annual Meeting of the Population Association of America, Washington, DC, March 28, 2011).
3 Although there were no official data published by the North Korean government, international aid agencies reported 230 deaths from cholera in 1995. In 2001, malaria peaked with 300,000 cases, and the prevalence of tuberculosis reached 220 cases per 10,000, from 38 cases in 1993. Jinhyouk Kim, "History of Epidemics in North Korea, 1945–2000," *Yonsei Journal of Medical History* 20 (2017): 79–81.
4 Shenyu Li et al., "Status of Intestinal Helminthic Infections of Borderline Residents in North Korea," *The Korean Journal of Parasitology* 44 (2006): 265.
5 Sunghwa Shin et al., "Serological Study on Human Parasite Infection in North Korea," *Seoul National University Unification Study Grant Reports* (2004): 1–2.
6 Paragonimiasis is a food-borne parasitic disease caused by *Paragonimus Westermani*. It is often referred to as lung fluke or lung diastema. This was endemic in East Asia, causing significant morbidity and mortality among people who consume raw crustaceans and freshwater fish.
7 Soon-young Ra, *Pediseutoma [Paragonimaisis]* (Pyongyang: Gungnipchulpansa, 1955).
8 Sun-won Hong, *Chosŏn pogŏnsa [History of Public Health in Korea]* (Pyongyang: Kwahak, Paekkwa Sajŏn Ch'ulp'ansa, 1981), 580.
9 Sahoe Kwahagwŏn Yŏksa Yŏnguso, *Chosŏn chŏnsa [History of Korea] Vol 29* (Pyongyang: Kwahak Paekkwa Sajŏn Chonghap Ch'ulpansa, 1981), 384.

10 These orders include Cabinet Order No. 9,F "On Organization and Implementation of Paragonimiasis Prevention and Treatment Measures" on February 9, 1955,
and Cabinet Decision No. 52, "On the Development of Sanitation Work as a Mass
Movement" on May 4, 1958. KCNA (Korean Central News Agency), *Chosŏn
chungang yŏn'gam (1956) [Korean Year Book]* (Pyongyang: KCNA. 1956), 472;
KCNA, *Chosŏn chungang yŏn'gam (1958) [Korean Year Book]* (Pyongyang: KCNA,
1958), 138.

11 Dracunculiasis is a parasitic disease caused by the Guinea worm, *Dracunculus med-
inensis*, and transmitted by freshwater crustaceans. When infected, adult worms
form boils on the skin for releasing the eggs, often in the lower extremities. During
this stage, the boils cause pain and a burning sensation. Repeated infection leads to
severe arthritis and lowers work ability. Litvinov S. K., "How the USSR Rid Itself
of Dracunculiasis," *World Health Forum* 12 (1991): 218–219.

12 Chosŏn Nodongdang Ch'ulp'ansa, *Inmin ŭi ŏbŏi [Father of the People] Vol 4*
(Pyongyang: Chosŏn Nodongdang Ch'ulp'ansa, 1975), 460–462; Hong, *Chosŏn
pogŏnsa*, 577–580; Sahoe Kwahagwŏn Yŏksa Yŏnguso, *Chosŏn chŏnsa Vol 29*,
384–386.

13 Chosŏn Nodongdang Ch'ulp'ansa, *Inmin ŭi ŏbŏi Vol 4* (Pyongyang: Chosŏn
Nodongdang Ch'ulp'ansa, 1975); Sun-won Hong, *Chosŏn pogŏnsa* (Pyongyang:
Kwahak, Paekkwa Sajŏn Ch'ulp'ansa, 1981); Sahoe Kwahagwŏn Yŏksa Yŏnguso,
Chosŏn chŏnsa Vol 29 (Pyongyang: Kwahak Paekkwa Sajŏn Chonghap Ch'ulpansa,
1981).

14 Jinhyouk Kim, "The Construction of Epidemic Prevention-Hygiene Systems and
the Development of 'the People's Consciousness' in North Korea (1945~1950),"
The Journal of Korean History 167 (2014): 247–287; Song-bong Lee, "North
Korea's Construction of Health Care System and Its Characteristics," *The Korean
Journal of Unification Affairs* 21 (2009): 323–357; Sang-ik Hwang, *North Korean
Health Care System During the Formative Period of Socialism in the 1950s* (Seoul:
Seoul National University Press, 2006).

15 Ok-ryun Moon, *Health System and Health Coverage in North Korea* (Seoul: Korean
National Health Insurance Agency, 1989); Jong-hwa Byun, *Comparative study
between the health systems of South and North Korea* (Seoul: KIHASA, 1993); Hong,
Chosŏn pogŏnsa; Hwang, *North Korean Health Care System*.

16 Tae-sup Lee, *Kim Il-sung Leadership* (Seoul: Deullyeok, 2001), 203.

17 Junho Jung, and Ock-joo Kim, "A Social History of Ascariasis in the 1960s Korea:
From a Norm to a Shameful Disease," *Korean Journal of Medical History* 25
(2016): 168.

18 David Grove, *A History of Human Helminthology* (Oxon: CABI International,
1990), 169–170.

19 Sun Huh, "Parasitic Diseases as the Cause of Death of Prisoners of War during the
Korean War (1950–1953)," *The Korean Journal of Parasitology* 52 (2014):
335–337.

20 Inmin pogŏn, "Diseutoma yebangsoreul chajaseo(pyeongbukdo hyangsangun)
[Report on Paragonimiasis Prevention Center]," *Inmin pogŏn[People's Public
Health]*, January, 1959, 58.

21 Ra, *Pediseutoma*, 41.

22 Ibid., 47–59.

23 Moon-bin Lim, "Noe diseutomajeunge gwanhayeo (1) [On Cerebral Paragonimi-
asis]," *Chosŏn ŭihak* 7~8 (1958): 11.

24 Inmin pogŏn, "Diseutoma yebangsoreul," 58.

25 Jiyoung Park et al., "Cerebral paragonimiasis and Bo Sung Sim's hemispherectomy
in Korea in 1950s–1960s," *Korean Journal of Medical History* 20 (2011): 132.

26 Tae-hwang Kim, "Pe diseutoma yeokageseoui myeot gaji munje [Some problems
on epidemiology of paragonimiasis]," *Inmin pogŏn*, September 1958, 27.

27 Soon-young Ra, "Uri naraeseoui pe diseutoma toechi bunyaeseo dalseonghan seonggwa [Accomplishment of Paragonimus eradication in our country]," *Chosŏn ŭihak [Korean Journal of Medicine]* 5 (1962): 43.

28 Jung-gyun Joo, *Hangukgisaengchunghagui hansegi [A Century of Korean Parasitology]* (Seoul: Gukjemunhwa, 1986).

29 Young-hoon Park, *Inche gisaengchunghak [Human Parasitology]* (Pyungyang: Godeunggyoyukdoseo chulpansa, 1961), 41.

30 Ra, *Pediseutoma*, 41–43.

31 Sung-chan Lee, "Dangui ttatteuthan baeryeoe bodapagetda(diseutoma jeungeul wanchihan gippeum) [I will repay the Party's warm care (Joy of curing paragonimiasis)]," *Wisaeng munhwa [Hygiene Culture]*, August, 1959, 26.

32 Sung-soon Joo, "Pediseutoma cheongsane gwanhan yeongu [Research on paragonimiasis eradication]," *Chosŏn ŭihak* 7~8 (1958), 19.

33 Chosŏn Nodongdang Ch'ulp'ansa, *Inmin ŭi ŏbŏi*, 74–79.

34 Hwang, North Korean Health Care System, 80–81.

35 Inmin pogŏn, "Diseutomawaui tujaengeseo sogeukseongeul geukbokaja [Overcome passiveness in struggle for paragonimiasis eradication]," *Inmin pogŏn* October 1958, 71.

36 Soon-hyung Lee, "Short History of Korean Society for Parasitology," *The Korean Journal of Parasitology* 17 (1979): 185–186.

37 Approximately 5 to 10 articles were published on Paragonimiasis in the Korean Peninsula from 1916 to late 1930s, ranging from clinical case reports to diagnostics and therapeutics. Also, there were numbers of articles on ecology of the disease, focusing on animal reservoir hosts and behaviors of intermediate hosts. Hyungsik Yoo. *History of Medical Research in Modern Korea, 1910~1945* (Seoul: Korean Institute of Medicine, 2011), 285–294.

38 Kyu-hwan Shin, "Research on endemic diseases and Japanese colonial rule: focusing on the emetine poisoning accident in Yeongheung and Haenam counties in 1927," *Korean Journal of Medical History* 18 (2009): 176–177.

39 Ra, *Pediseutoma*.

40 Ibid., 83.

41 Zhong Hui-lan (1901–1987) was one of the founders of tropical medicine in China. He discovered new species of *Paragonimus, Paragonimus sichuanensis*, in Sichuan, 1962. Gan Shaobo, "Introduction to Professor ZHONG Hui-lan, One of the Founders of Tropical Medicine in China," *China Tropical Medicine* 9 (2009): 399.

42 Ra, *Pediseutoma*.

43 Shin, "Research on Endemic Diseases," 184.

44 А. Бердыев, "Полина Андреевна Петрищева и значение её трудов в развитии паразитологии(к 100-летию со дня рождения)[Polina Andreevna Petrishcheva and the significance of her works in the development of parasitology (to the 100th anniversary of the birth)]" *Паразитология[Parasitology]* 33 (1999): 1.

45 Jinhyouk Kim and Mira Moon, "The Socialist Camp's North Korean Medical Support and Exchange (1945–1958): Between Learning from the Soviet Union and Independent Course," *Korean Journal of Medical History* 28 (2019): 144–154.

46 Skrjabin (1878–1972) was a parasitologist in the Soviet Union, often referred to as the father of helminthology in Russia. Skrjabin graduated from the Yuriev Veterinary Institute in 1905, worked as a veterinarian, and was appointed as a professor of parasitology at the University of Novocherkassk. K. M. Ryzhikov, "An Appreciation of Academician K. I. Skrjabin, Founder of the Soviet Helminthological School, on the Occasion of the Centenary of His Birth," *Journal of Helminthology* 52 (1978): 171–172; Герой Социалистического Труда [Hero of Socialist Labor]. "Скрябин Константин Иванович[Skryabin Konstantin Ivanovich]." Accessed September 1, 2021. http://www.warheroes.ru/hero/hero.asp?Hero_id=11440

47 After Skrjabin was appointed as a professor, he organized a parasitological expedition to identify human and animal parasites, with descriptions of the ecological characteristics in the entire ecosystem of the Soviet region. The expedition, which was first launched in 1919 and continued with 335 expeditions until 1966, discovered more than 900 new parasites and 50 new human parasites. К. И. Скрябин, "Основные этапы развития гельминтологии в СССР за 50 лет [The main development of helminthology in the USSR for 50 years]," *Паразитология[Parasitology]* 1 (1967): 356–358.

48 Ministry of Health, *Dracunculiasis Eradication in Uzbekistan: Country Report* (Geneva: World Health Organization, 1999): 13–15.

49 Герой Социалистического Труда. "Скрябин Константин Иванович."

50 Ministry of Health, *Dracunculiasis Eradication*, 26–29.

51 Марк Поповский, *Тот, кто спорил. Повесть о Леониде Исаеве. Люди среди людей Повести [The one who argued. The story of Leonid Isaev. People among people Tale]* (Детская литература, 1972).

52 Ministry of Health, *Dracunculiasis Eradication*, 26–29.

53 Скрябин, "Основные этапы развития гельминтологии," 368.

54 Report to assembly in 1944 was later published as "Sanitary and economic significance of helminthiasis in the national economy of the USSR and the problem of their elimination (Санитарно-экономическаязначимость гельминтозов в народном хозяй-стве СССР и проблема их ликвидации)".

55 К. И. Скрябин, *Девастация в борьбе с гельминтозами и другими болезнями человека и животных [Devastation in the fight against helminthiases and other human and animal diseases]* (Изд-во Кирг. ф-ла АН СССР, 1947).

56 Ra, *Pediseutoma*, 41.

57 Ryzhikov, "An Appreciation of Academician K. I. Skrjabin," 171–172.

58 Ra, *Pediseutoma*, 120–122.

59 Ibid., 108.

60 In the ideological struggle (reeducation) for old intelligentsia in the health care sector between 1956 and 1961, the emphasis on treatment over prevention was heavily criticized as bourgeois ideology. This was characteristic of Soviet medicine. North Korea adopted this idea for multiple reasons. First, a scarcity of resources limited the use of drugs. Second, as means of ideological struggle, this substituted the older generation of doctors trained in the colonial period who were more interested in research with the new generation of "red" doctors willing to work in the field. For more details, see Junho Jung, Minkyu Kim and Ock-joo Kim, "Creating the Red Health Warrior: Ideological Struggle in North Korea's Health Care Sector, 1956–1961," *The Korean Journal for the History of Science* 40 (2018): 425–478.

61 Ra, *Pediseutoma*, 108.

62 Ibid., 158.

63 Ibid.

64 Miriam Gross, *Farewell to the God of Plague: Chairman Mao's Campaign to Deworm China* (California: University of California Press, 2016), 21–25.

65 Zhihua Shen and Yafeng Xia, *A Misunderstood Friendship: Mao Zedong, Kim Il-sung, and Sino-North Korean Relations, 1949–1976* (Columbia University Press, 2020), 77–86.

66 Jegeun Chi, "First 50 Years of Department of Pathology Seoul National University College of Medicine," *Korean Journal of Medical History* 5 (1996): 7.

67 Sung-soon Joo, "Pheytisuthoma chengsan saepeyse etun myechkaci kyenghem [Some lessons learned from Paragonimiasis eradication program]," *Inmin pogŏn*, September 1957, 12.

68 Schistosomiasis is a disease transmitted through contacting water contaminated by juvenile parasites, with the intermate hosts of snails similar to paragonimiasis. It is often referred to as "snail fever," causing high fever, and chronic infection leads to

liver failure. It was a major endemic disease in river areas of China since antiquity. Gross, *Farewell to the God of Plague*, 7–12.

69 The village was located in Sinsanggun, Hamgyeongnamdo on the eastern side of North Korea. It was in a mountain region, with more than 100 households and many migrants. Joo, "Pheytisuthoma chengsan," 12.

70 Ra, *Pediseutoma*, 82.

71 Ibid., 82–85.

72 Chang-su Choi, "Diseutoma toechi saeobeseo eodeun gyeongheom [Lessons learned from paragonimiasis eradication project]," *Inmin pogŏn*, October 1960, 28.

73 Ra, *Pediseutoma*, 93.

74 KCNA, *Chosŏn chungang yŏn'gam (1956)*, 472.

75 Ra, *Pediseutoma*, 134.

76 KCNA, *Chosŏn chungang yŏn'gam (1956)*, 127.

77 Ra, *Pediseutoma*, 45–46.

78 Chosŏn Nodongdang Ch'ulp'ansa, *Inmin ŭi ŏbŏi*, 75.

79 Inmin pogŏn. "Diseutoma yebangsoreul chajaseo (pyeongbukdo hyangsangun) [Report on Paragonimiasis Prevention Center]," *Inmin pogŏn*, January 1959, 58.

80 KCNA, *Chosŏn chungang yŏn'gam (1957)* [Korean Year Book] (Pyongyang: KCNA. 1957), 103.

81 Ra, *Pediseutoma*, 119–123.

82 Ryang-mo Han, "Gisaengseong geosebeobe uihan diseutoma golbaengi somyeol daechaege gwanhan yeongu[Eliminating Paragonimiasis snails through parasitic castration]," *Chosŏn ŭihak* 5 (1962): 12.

83 Ra, *Pediseutoma*, 46.

84 Yunha Yoon, Ock-joo Kim and Junho Jung, "Hygiene and the Making of the Socialist Lifestyle: Reconstruction of the People through the Hygiene Culture Project in North Korea in the late 1950s," *The Korean Journal for the History of Science* 40 (2018): 513–514.

85 Dong-pal Lee, "Diseutoma junggan sukju bangmyeol saeobeseo eodeun gyeongheom(pyeongbukdo changseonggun je1diseutoma yebangso) [Lessons learned from paragonimiasis intermediate host(1 Paragonimiasis prevention center of Chang-sung]," *Inmin pogŏn*, April, 1959, 33–35.

86 Rodong Sinmun, "Cisuthomauy yeypang taychayk [Preventive measures on Paragonimiasis]," *Rodong Sinmun*, April 27, 1957.

87 Inmin pogŏn, "Diseutoma yebangsoreul chajaseo(pyeongbukdo hyangsangun) [Report on Paragonimiasis Prevention Center]," *Inmin pogŏn*, January, 1959, 58.

88 Junho Jung and Ock-joo Kim, "A Social History of Ascariasis in the 1960s Korea: From a Norm to a Shameful Disease," *Korean Journal of Medical History* 25 (2016): 201–202.

89 Joo, "Pheytisuthoma chengsan saepeyse," 12.

90 Yoon et al, "Hygiene and the Making of the Socialist Lifestyle," 514.

91 Joo, "Pheytisuthoma chengsan saepeyse," 12.

92 Dong-man Seo. *Pukchosŏn sahoejuŭi ch'eje sŏngnipsa, 1945–1961 [Formation of North Korean Socialist System, 1945–1961]* (Paju: Sŏnin, 2005), 760–764.

93 Central Committee of Workers' Party of Korea. "1956nyeondo joseonnodongdangjungangwiwonhoe jeonwonhoeui·jeongchi·sangmu·jojigwiwonhoe gyeoljeongjip [Decisions from Organization Committee of Politics, Standing Committee of Central Committee of Workers' Party of Korea 1956]," in *Historical Materials for North Korea Relationship*, ed. National Institute of Korean History (Gwacheon: National Institute of Korean History), 789–795.

94 Lee, *Kim Il-sung Leadership*, 68–69.

95 KCNA, *Chosŏn chungang yŏn'gam(1958)*, 138.

96 Jong-ryul Lee, *Bogeonjojikak [Organizing Public Health]* (Pyongyang: Godeung-gyoyukdoseochulpansa, 1962), 75.

97 Joo, "Pediseutoma cheongsane gwanhan yeongu," 20.

98 Ibid., 17–21.

99 Joseonnodongdangchulpansa, *Gimilseongjeojakjip 12* [Writings of Kim Il-sung 12] (Pyongyang: Joseonnodongdangchulpansa, 1981), 246.

100 KCNA, *Chosŏn chungang yŏn'gam (1959) [Korean Year Book]* (Pyongyang: KCNA, 1959), 81.

101 Ho-je Kang, *History of science and technology in North Korea* (Paju: Sŏnin, 2007), 213–214.

102 KCNA, *Chosŏn chungang yŏn'gam (1959)*, 81.

103 The method of implementing a specialized center for a specific disease in North Korea may reflect the earlier experience in China. During the early 1950s, China incorporated a schistosomiasis eradication program into the broader public health program and developed generalized epidemic disease prevention stations. This attempt was rather unsuccessful as resources were diverged among many programs within the station and lost focus along the way. In November 1955, Mao instructed to develop an independent national program for schistosomiasis eradication and effectively separated the activities from general sanitation programs. Gross, *Farewell to the God of Plague*, 23–25.

104 Hwang, *North Korean Health Care System*, 87.

105 Leonard Bruce-Chwatt, "Malaria Research and Eradication in the USSR: A Review of Soviet Achievements in the Field of Malariology," *Bulletin of the World Health Organization* 21 (1959): 737.

106 Zhihua Shen and Yafeng Xia, *A Misunderstood Friendship*, 126–136.

107 Ra, *Pediseutoma*, 108–109.

108 Chul-soo Lee, *Laws of healthcare in North Korea* (Seoul: Gyechungmunhwasa, 2006), 248.

109 KCNA, *Chosŏn chungang yŏn'gam (1959)*, 81–83.

110 Inmin pogŏn, "Hangdiseutoma tujaengeul wihan jeonmun il'gun gangseup jin-haeng [Special health workers training for anti-paragonimiasis]," *Inmin pogŏn* October, 1958, 21.

111 Inmin pogŏn, "Diseutoma yebang chiryo jeonmun il'gun mit jungdeungbogeon il'gun yangseong saeobeul seonggwajeogeuro bojanghal jochireul ganggu [Consideration of effective training of specialized primary and secondary health workers in paragonimiasis prevention center]," *Inmin pogŏn*, September, 1958, 74.

112 KCNA, *Chosŏn chungang yŏn'gam (1959)*, 81.

113 Hong, *Chosŏn pogŏnsa*, 578.

114 Ra, *Pediseutoma*, 51.

115 Inmin pogŏn, "Sangbannyeon jungeuro diseutomaneun eopseojinda: gaeseong jigunae inmindeul diseutoma bangmyeore jeokgeuk Dongwon [Paragonimiasis will be gone in first half of this year: mobilizing people of Gaesung to eradicate the disease]," *Inmin pogŏn*, June, 1959, 56.

116 Inmin pogŏn, "Gonghwagugui jeonche bogeon ilkkundeulgwa jeonguk bogeon ilkkun hoeui chamgaja dongjideurege (joseon rodongdang jungangwiwonhoee-seo bonaen pyeonji) [To all health worker in the republic and to all participants in National Health Workers Meeting (Letter from Worker's Party Korea)]," *Inmin pogŏn*, May, 1959, 2–4.

117 Joseonnodongdangchulpansa, *Gimilseongjeojakjip 12*, 246.

118 Jung et al., "Creating the Red Health Warrior," 438–440.

119 Ibid., 475–476.

120 Inmin pogŏn, "Gak uihak daehak mit uihak jeonmun hakgyo haksaengdeurui wisaeng gongjageseo jaengchwihan binnaneun seonggwa [Shining achievement

of each medical school student in public health activities]," *Inmin pogŏn*, September 1958, 70–71.

121 Inmin pogŏn, "Galsugireul riyonghayeo gajae, golbaengi jabireul gunjungjeok undongeuro jeongae [Collecting snails and crayfish during dry season as public activity, from Pyungbuk, Chang-sung]," *Inmin pogŏn*, October 1958, 47.

122 Ra, *Pediseutoma*, 125.

123 Lee, "Diseutoma junggan sukju," 26.

124 Jang-han Park, "Diseutoma junggan sukju bangmyeol saeobeseo hyeongmyeongjeok daechaegi yogudoenda [Call for revolutionary measures in paragonimiasis intermediate host eradication]," *Inmin pogŏn*, 1959, 44.

125 Ra, *Pediseutoma*, 115.

126 Wisaeng munhwa, "Orireul riyonghayeo golbaengi jabi[Catching snails with ducks]," *Wisaeng munhwa*, July 1959, 23.

127 Park, *Inche gisaengchunghak*, 49.

128 Ra, "Uri naraeseoui pe diseutoma toechi," 44.

129 Ra, *Pediseutoma*, 114.

130 Chosŏn Nodongdang Ch'ulp'ansa, *Inmin ŭi ŏbŏi*, 74–79.

131 KCNA, *Chosŏn chungang yŏn'gam (1959)*, 81.

132 Yoon et al., "Hygiene and the Making of the Socialist Lifestyle," 501–525.

133 Hong, *Chosŏn pogŏnsa*, 535.

134 Sung-chan Lee, "Dangui ttatteuthan baeryeoe bodapagetda(diseutoma jeungeul wanchihan gippeum) [I will repay the Party's warm care (Joy of curing paragonimiasis)]," *Wisaeng munhwa*, August, 1959, 26.

135 Park, *Inche gisaengchunghak*, 41.

136 Lee, *Bogeonjojikak*, 81.

137 The exact date of the eradication is rather questionable, as it usually takes a few years to declare eradication of the endemic disease with extensive follow-ups. Considering the limited ability to treat active cases during the 1950s, the adult parasite may have survived in its asymptomatic carriers for a while. It would be safe to assume that the eventual eradication of the paragonimiasis took a few more years than was declared by the North Korean government.

138 Park, *Inche gisaengchunghak*, 10.

139 Sahoe Kwahagwŏn Yŏksa Yŏnguso, *Chosŏn chŏnsa Vol 29*, 388.

140 Dora Vargha, "Technical assistance and socialist international health: Hungary, the WHO and the Korean War," *History and Technology* 36 (2020): 409–411.

141 Kee Park, Younghan Roh, Owen Lee-Park and Sophie Park, "History of neurosurgery in Democratic People's Republic of Korea," *World Neurosurgery* 84 (2015): 855–856; Dumitru Mohan, "Dr. Lenke Horvath (1917–1991): Creator of Pediatric Neurosurgery in Romania," *World Neurosurgery* 88 (2016): 652–653.

142 Kang, *History of Science and Technology in North Korea*, 131–132.

143 Byung-nam Lee, "Jeonhu 3gaenyeon bogeon saeop chonghwawa 1957nyeondo dangmyeon gwaeobe daehayeo(jeonhu 3gaenyeon bogeon saeop chonghwa hoeuieseoui bogo) [Summary of the postwar three-year health project and current tasks in 1957 (Report at the postwar three-year health project summary meeting)]," *Inmin pogŏn*, April 1957, 13.

144 Ho-rim Lee, "8·15 haebang 13junyeoneul majeumyeo [Celebrating the 13th anniversary of the 8.15 liberation]," *Chosŏn ŭihak*. 7~8 (1958): 2–4.

145 Zhihua Shen and Yafeng Xia, *A Misunderstood Friendship*, 77–79.

3 Toward Economic Growth

The Development of Public Health Activities in South Korea from 1961 to 1988

Park Yunjae

Introduction

In 1961, a military coup took place in South Korea. The brief experiment with democracy was over. In terms of public health, however, the coup meant a new beginning. To achieve economic growth—proclaimed as the main cause of the military coup—the military government began to build a public health system, which was essential for securing people's health. Unhealthy citizens could not constitute the strong labor force necessary for economic growth. The military government began to lay out public health programs in conjunction with economic development plans.

Ensuring health was not only a goal of the government, however. The Korean people did not show clear resistance to joining public health projects promoted by the government. Without the cooperation of the people, carrying out large-scale projects, such as parasite eradication or anti-tuberculosis efforts, would have been almost impossible. According to the memories of people who joined these projects, these citizens were sincere, ardent, and occasionally rash. This could be called a cooperative period between the government and the people.

If this was indeed the case, I would like to examine what was behind the cooperation. People could be forced to join the projects, but if they agreed with the goal (promoting health), they could also willingly participate. What made the Korean people contribute their time and effort to these massive projects? Another question I would like to raise concerns the projects' results. The projects could be evaluated as successes. The egg-positive rate of parasites, which was 84.3% in 1972, dropped to 3.8% by 1992. Tuberculosis infection in children between 0 and 4 years old decreased to 4.9% in 1980 from 10.2% in 1965. The most dramatic change was in population growth. The national average of 5.8 children in 1961 dropped to 2.6 in 1979. To call this success is not an exaggeration.

Medical supply centers tell a different story, however. After the 1960s, the Korean government endeavored to strengthen the basis of public health centers and resolve the problem of doctorless villages. However, the share of public hospitals in the field of medical treatment was decreasing. It is necessary

DOI: 10.4324/9781003318163-4

to ask what the result of this situation was and think about the direction in which that result has led the Korean public health system.

Another issue I would like to examine is how international support influenced public health activities in South Korea and what this meant. The World Health Organization (WHO), UNICEF, and the Overseas Technology Cooperation Agency (OTCA) of Japan inaugurated anti-epidemic projects and supported a tuberculosis survey and an anti-parasite program. Without financial and technical support from international organizations, such nationwide programs could not have materialized. The reason why international organizations supported South Korea may have something to do with the Cold War. Generally, the Korean Peninsula was estimated to be at the forefront of the Cold War after the Korean War. This chapter attempts to find the connection between the support of international organizations and the establishment of a public health system in South Korea.

There is little research on this topic in English. One relevant study is *Reconstructing Bodies* by John Dimoia.[1] His work covers family planning and anti-parasite campaigns. According to Dimoia, the state was able to protect the bodies of Koreans through nationwide projects, largely due to the influence of Western medicine. As a result, he argues, South Koreans came to make medicine of their own along with the associated physical interventions, such as physical examinations, injections, surgeries, and autopsies.[2] My work investigates these topics more comprehensively, dealing with the laws and systems related to the changes in and development of the public health system in South Korea. My work will, I hope, identify the trajectory and dynamics of the public health system in South Korea.

The Development of National Anti-Infectious Disease Projects and Public–Private Partnerships

The Establishment of Public Health Centers

After the liberation, South Korea was under the rule of a U.S. military government for three years, so the United States exerted a strong influence over South Korea. Public health centers in South Korea were established to achieve the ideal of preventive medicine formulated in the United States before World War II. The American system of health care was notable for its division of labor between the state, which took on the task of public health administration, and private practitioners, who provided medical services.[3] Public health centers in South Korea, however, were not able to realize the ideal of preventive medicine. The shortage of medical supplies was severe, so public health centers could only function as small dispensaries.

In 1946, South Korea saw the first establishment of a public health center, which followed the plans made at the 1937 Intergovernmental Conference of Far-Eastern Countries on Rural Health in Bandung. The public health center was intended to provide primary healthcare services in Ceylon first. It began as part of the Rockefeller Foundation's hookworm eradication campaign in the region.[4] The Korean War gave a chance to increase the number of public health centers. As the threat posed by the Korean War of spreading epidemic diseases increased, public health dispensaries devoted to anti-epidemic activities began to appear, and their number reached 520 during the Korean War. In July 1951, public health dispensaries were reorganized as public health centers that put theoretically more effort into public health activities. This measure was taken with the intention of establishing public health centers nationwide.[5]

It was recommended that public health centers should be progressively transformed until they could carry out all local health work, both environmental and personal; they would also undertake some curative work, but this would be secondary to their main preventive function. However, the reality was different. None of the public health centers conducted any kind of preliminary health surveys in their assigned areas. The main challenge that public health centers faced was low-quality medical staff. Not a single medical officer in charge of a center had taken an elementary course of postgraduate training in public health.[6]

A full-scale attempt to strengthen public health centers began in the 1960s. The law on public health centers was completely amended in 1961. The revision of the law aimed to center the role of public health centers around the propagation of preventive medicine. These centers were now in charge of all duties of technical administration related to health and hygiene, as well as the guidance and supervision of public medical doctors, who were previously managed by cities, counties, and districts. The revised law allowed for more localized operations and supervision. This revision "laid the foundation for epoch-making development by strengthening medical preventive measures for disease and overall health administration."[7]

The revision of the law led to a reduction in public health centers. The number of public health centers, which had exceeded 500 in the 1950s, was reduced to 189 by 1963. Given that there were 140 counties nationwide in 1960, an average of only 1.35 health centers were left for each county.

The system was renovated—but public health centers were in bad shape. As a result of a lack of various medical instruments, facilities, equipment, and administrative and technical staff, the centers were unable to perform their original duties. In terms of personnel, out of 217 public health centers in the early 1980s, only 172 had overseers. The recruitment rate was 79%. Above all, there was a large pay gap with private medical institutions: at best, public employees made 40% of what private medical institutions offered and, at worst, only 16%. Securing excellent medical personnel was very difficult in these conditions.[8]

Concerns about the future of public health centers continued. One desire was that public health centers remain primary medical institutions focused on preventive medicine. The government made several attempts to ensure this. For instance, it placed public health nurses in charge of comprehensive health projects, such as health prevention, education, and nutrition improvement.[9] However, Users perceived public health centers as being in charge of just vaccination or anti-epidemic activity or as refuges used by the poor.[10]

Although several problems were pointed out, it is clear that the public health center was an important institution that contributed to the health and longevity of Koreans. Public health centers "excluded Koreans from the 'parasite kingdom', established rules for small numbers of children through family planning, and showed the possibility of eradicating tuberculosis through tuberculosis management."[11]

The Multilateral Tuberculosis Eradication Project

Tuberculosis has been a priority among infectious diseases for a long time in Korea. During the colonial period, tuberculosis patients who should have been hospitalized were estimated to number about 40,000 out of a population of 20 million. Tuberculosis was the disease with the largest number of patients. After the liberation, this number increased. In the 1950s, a million people were estimated to suffer from tuberculosis. Of these, about half were estimated to need treatment.[12]

National measures for treating tuberculosis patients were prepared in the 1960s, and they delegated key responsibilities to public health centers. In 1962, as the Public Health Center Act was revised and promulgated, tuberculosis control projects were developed through public health centers.[13] Another factor was foreign support. In 1961, South Korea and the WHO signed an aid agreement on tuberculosis control projects. As a result, the South Korean government launched a national tuberculosis control program. In 1962, financial support from UNICEF was set in motion.[14] Prior to the WHO's assistance, tuberculosis control in Korea had been limited to basic administrative activities and intermittent vaccination campaigns by the government.[15]

In 1962, public health centers initiated patient registration and treatment. Across the country, 189 public health centers, 670 public doctor clinics, and 59 designated clinics participated in the home treatment of registered patients.[16] In 1963, tuberculosis management doctors were assigned to every province except Jeju Island. They participated in technical guidance and planning of all tuberculosis projects in their area.[17] With their oversight, it was possible to "establish the foundation of a tuberculosis management project."[18]

In 1963, the Korean Tuberculosis Association dispatched tuberculosis management personnel, who had undergone regular training, to 189 public health centers across the country. In other words, a private organization dispatched personnel to work for government organizations.[19] This arrangement of delegating public tuberculosis control activities to voluntary associations was a temporary measure at a time when the government still did not have the administrative capacity to pursue full-scale anti-tuberculosis activities.[20] It was not until 1967 that management responsibility for these individuals was transferred to the government.

The first nationwide tuberculosis survey was conducted in 1965. The Korean Tuberculosis Association initiated this survey with administrative support from the government, technical support from the WHO, and material support from UNICEF. Specifically, the tuberculosis infection rate, the prevalence of pulmonary tuberculosis on X-rays, and tuberculosis bacillus–positive rate, was investigated in local residents according to gender, age, and city and county. This survey was the third largest in the world after those of Japan and Taiwan.[21] Subsequently, the National Tuberculosis Survey was conducted by selecting a sample area to represent the whole country every five years.

In 1967, the government enacted the Tuberculosis Prevention Act. Its main purpose was to enable the national and local governments to prevent tuberculosis and provide adequate medical care for patients. Those subject to medical examination were obliged to take the examination within a designated period. It also established a tuberculosis control review committee and raised money for the Christmas Seal.[22] In Korea, the first Christmas Seal was issued in 1932 by Western missionary doctor Sherwood Hall, who got the idea while he stayed in the United States on furlough.[23] In 1967, through the reorganization of the Ministry of Public Health and Social Affairs, the Tuberculosis Division became independent from the Chronic Disease Division within the Health Bureau.[24] Throughout the 1960s, a government-level legal system and organization devoted to tuberculosis were systematically formed.

The tuberculosis project, which had been in full swing since the 1960s, yielded results. In those between the ages of 0 and 29, the tuberculosis infection rate decreased from 44.5% in 1965 to 41.7% in 1980. The ratios of decreases in the age ranges of 0 to 4, 5 to 9, and 10 to 14 for the same period were 10.2% to 4.9%, 33.7% to 12.6%, and 69.5% to 32.1%, respectively.[25]

The prevention of tuberculosis represented by BCG and progress in treatment through the introduction of new drugs helped reduce the disease. Another noteworthy measure to this end was the establishment of a tuberculosis management system led by the government. In particular, public health centers played an important role in reducing tuberculosis. The public health center acted as "the center of all tuberculosis projects."[26] Progress in tuberculosis projects, such as tuberculosis testing and patient registration and management, was linked to the expansion of these centers. Furthermore, the government accumulated basic data to support management projects through nationwide surveys. These included a nationwide sputum examination, X-ray examination, and tuberculosis survey conducted every five years.[27]

The Parasite Eradication Project

Parasites used to be one of the most common ailments in Korea. According to a survey conducted by the government in 1948, more than nine out of ten people were infected with a parasite.[28] This astronomical infection rate was due to inadequate toilet facilities and the use of human fertilizer. Night soil had long been the primary source of fertilizer in Korea. Parasites that emerged from human feces reentered the body through food. It was a vicious circle.

A full-scale parasite eradication project began in the 1960s. The establishment of the Korea Association on Eradication of Parasites in 1964 was an important opportunity. In 1965, the government appointed the deputy mayor or deputy governor as the branch head of the Korea Association on Eradication of Parasites and the head of the provincial health and social affairs bureau as the deputy head.[29] Civil servants were assigned to this new private organization. As a result, while the organization was still officially private, it became a private–government hybrid de facto.

In 1966, the Parasitic Disease Prevention Act was enacted to prevent and eradicate parasitic diseases. At that time, Korea and Japan were the only places in East and South Asia where such laws were enacted.[30] The law stipulated that those in an area prone to parasitic diseases and who engaged in occupations that involved frequent contact with the public due to the nature of their work should undergo examination and treatment at least once a year. It also required that school principals at each level inspect and treat every student for parasite infection at least twice a year. Furthermore, this law designated the Korea Association on Eradication of Parasites as an institution that conducts research and prevention projects on parasites.[31] With the enactment of this law, the union between the government and the private sector was legally confirmed.

In 1969, the Korea Association on Eradication of Parasites was introduced by the government and began conducting parasite testing and deworming programs for all elementary, middle, and high school students across the country twice a year, in spring and autumn.[32] Students were forced to provide a feces sample to their teachers twice a year. If they were found to be infected by parasites, they had to take a vermicide in front of their colleagues. The enactment of this law was evaluated as "a comprehensive declaration of war on parasites," as if, "at least in elementary, middle and high schools, a total mobilization order was issued."[33] The scope of mobilization was later expanded to laborers, soldiers, and so on.

The act was promulgated and the students were tested, but the enforcement body was not prepared. There was a shortage of trained manpower and inspection equipment capable of conducting group inspections.[34] At this time, cooperation from foreign countries was an important factor that made it possible to carry out projects such as inspection and deworming. In particular, cooperation with Japan was important after the renewal of diplomatic relations in 1965.

Japan provided testing equipment and medicine to the Korea Association on Eradication of Parasites between 1968 and 1972, the early stage of the project. With the introduction of new equipment and drugs, "inspection stations were completed in each province, and personnel for each field necessary for the project were deployed."[35] Around 1970, the cellophane thick smear technique, which was used for group testing in Japan, was applied. To elimi-nate the source of infection or reduce its intensity at the community level, speed, economy, and efficiency were important. The cellophane thick smear technique was "the most suitable method," given these criteria.[36] It played a major role in gathering biological samples in bulk, making "a great contribu-tion to the achievement of the goal of 0% parasites."[37]

Japan was also responsible for training the personnel in charge of the pro-ject. Parasitology experts and technical personnel from the OTCA provided training on parasitology.[38] Japan wanted to demonstrate the goodwill of a nation becoming an economic powerhouse in East Asia. The parasite manage-ment project conducted in Korea has been judged the most successful among the international cooperative projects supported by Japan.[39] If the tuberculosis project was carried out with the support of international organizations such as the WHO and UNICEF, the parasite eradication project is an example of Japan's more active support.

Korea also accepted Japanese group examination and group treatment methods. In 1971, the National Intestinal Parasite Infection Rate Survey was conducted by the Ministry of Public Health and Social Affairs and the Korea Association on Eradication of Parasites. This survey was conducted every five years, and the first survey was conducted in a total of 86 areas, including 46 urban and 40 rural areas.[40]

The impact of group examination and treatment was clear. According to the survey results, the egg-positive rate was 84.3% in 1971, 63.2% in 1976, 41.4% in 1981, 12.9% in 1986, and 3.8% in 1992. Roundworms also decreased from 54.9% in 1971 to 41.0% in 1976, 13.0% in 1981, 2.1% in 1986, and 0.3% in 1992. By 1992, the rate of most parasitic infections had dropped to less than 1%.[41]

The Korea Association on Eradication of Parasites, which led the project, pointed to examination as the biggest reason for the reduction of parasites. In particular, the group examination and the treatment of elementary, middle, and high school students conducted every spring and autumn contributed the most to the sharp drop in the infection rate. The annual number of people to be examined was 18 million, approximately 60% of the population in South Korea in the 1970s.[42]

The association's efforts were effective. This was not only because the target areas were scattered across the country but also because there were cases in which the target households were either absent or did not comply with the inspection. The people in charge carried out the investigation with "the deter-mination and mindset of 'you can do it.'" The government also actively sup-ported the project. As the government subsidized the inspection fee, large-scale inspections of elementary, middle, and high school students became possible. The fee was less than the cost of a single bus ride at that time, but in terms of the overall scale, it was "never a small amount."[43] School participation was also high. Schools became the central means through which the campaign con-ducted the majority of its collection activities. Principals, teachers, and students were "well aware of the significance and importance of group management."[44]

It could be said that the whole nation was sympathetic to the significance of the eradication of parasites. There was some passive resistance, such as students who accepted the medication offered but later disposed of it. However, there were few questions raised about the methods of sample gathering or the mass distribution of chemical remedies still in development.[45] The desire to achieve modernization and advancement was the background for people to participate in the parasite eradication project. The parasite retention rate was inversely proportional to cultural development, and to become an advanced country, the retention rate had to be lowered.[46]

However, the creation of a hygienic environment was also important. The parasite infection rate could be lowered by sanitizing human waste through the installation of flush toilets and improving sewage facilities. Economic growth was also necessary. The reduction of parasitic diseases was achieved as Korea grew economically and improved sanitation facilities and the surrounding environment.[47] Economic growth and the establishment of a sanitary environment were the fundamental background for the eradication of parasites.

Economic Development and Health

Family Planning Projects and Population Control

After the liberation and the Korean War, the population and fertility rate of South Korea rapidly increased. The main cause was the postwar baby boom. The population growth rate reached 3% per year. The total fertility rate in 1960 was 6.0%, continuing the high fertility rate of the 1940s.[48] It was thus necessary to curb population growth.

The prevention of communism was the international background for the family planning project to begin. Concerns that economic poverty could lead to political instability and communism were spreading around the United States. Population growth was a major obstacle to economic development, and it had been argued that population control was necessary for economic stability. Population growth in developing countries, such as South Korea, was a factor that threatened the world order centered on the United States during the Cold War.[49]

Economic growth was a direct trigger that sparked a concrete approach to the population problem in South Korea—namely, the family planning project. According to the Korea Association of Family Planning, solving the population problem was the path to economic growth, the improvement of living standards, and the realization of a welfare society. A "welfare society that achieves a national income of $1,000, which is the long-cherished dream of our people," could only be achieved by slowing the population growth rate to 1.3%.[50] Thus, family planning was regarded as an urgent economic problem rather than as a problem of public health.[51]

The direct impetus for starting a family planning project came, as with other national projects, from abroad. In November 1960, the International Planned Parenthood Federation dispatched George W. Cadbury and his wife to Korea as special representatives. They consulted with government and private officials about the launch of the family planning movement. As a result, the Korea Association of Family Planning was established in April 1961. It was the first organization in South Korea to make public the title of family planning.[52]

Most funding for the family planning project came from abroad as well. The Population Council (Rockefeller) and the Sweden International Development Authority prominently supported the project. The latter was involved with the distribution of the birth control pill. Visits by Koreans to Taichung, Taiwan, in 1963 provided access to a rich source of population data dating to the late nineteenth century as well as an opportunity for observation before the Koreans actively undertook their own project.[53]

The military government expanded the family planning project to the national level. In November 1961, the National Reconstruction Supreme Council passed the "Resolution of Family Planning Promotion." The idea was for the family planning project to be promoted as part of a five-year economic development plan guided by the belief that population growth would be an impediment to economic development. "It was an epoch-making day in the history of Korean population policy."[54] In June 1963, the government established the Maternal and Child Health Team in the Ministry of Public Health and Social Affairs as the central executive organization in charge of the family planning project.[55] It has been suggested that "the family planning project was based on a new conception of improving the economic fortunes of South Korea by establishing control over the population."[56]

Just as important as the central organization was the organizations that would actually implement the family planning project in each region. In 1962, the government set up family planning counseling centers at public health centers in 183 cities and counties across the country and dispatched midwives and nurses. This was the beginning of a nationwide family planning project. At that time, public health centers had 30 to 35 employees, of which more than half were in charge of family planning.[57] The main work of the public health center had been the control of tuberculosis, maternity, and childbirth until the start of family planning when it shifted focus to the family planning project.

In 1964, the government deployed family planning personnel in 1,473 towns and villages to strengthen sub-organizations at the municipal level. They were in charge of public awareness about family planning, home visits, and group guidance for contraceptive distribution. The family planning personnel changed the family planning project from a visitor-centered model to one based on home visits.[58] It was a more active method suitable for rural areas.[59]

The family planning project expanded to urban areas in the 1970s. In 1974, the hospital family planning project was implemented for urban, middle-class residents who used general hospitals. On the outskirts of Seoul, 10 family planning counseling centers were set up to provide contraceptive services to the poor in the city.[60]

In 1973, the Maternal and Child Health Act was enacted. Its purpose was to protect the lives and health of mothers and contribute to the improvement of public health by promoting the birth and rearing of healthy children. With the promulgation of this act, the permissible limits for abortion surgery were set, and it became possible to subsidize the expenses of family planning personnel.[61] Thus, 1973 was "a year in which a great milestone was drawn in the history of family planning projects."[62]

The first contraceptive methods supplied by the government were conventional ones, such as the diaphragm cycle, jellied effervescent tablets, condoms, and vasectomies. However, most conventional methods of contraception besides condoms were ineffective, so their distribution was soon halted.[63] Designed for rapid insertion into the female body, the loop represented the most recent attempt to provide a safe, inexpensive means of preventing pregnancy.

The loop, the representation of a new form of technology, had many advantages. It was economical and had few side effects. If there were severe side effects, it could be removed; if removed, pregnancy was possible again. As one observer put it, the "loop is the most effective, safe and acceptable method of contraception today."[64] However, the loop had a problem. After attachment, side effects appeared, such as bleeding and back pain. The loop also required a high degree of familiarity with its use. Thus, women began to stop wearing loops. Furthermore, the insertion procedure was not simple.[65] Despite the side effects, the loop was the most widely used method of birth control until the 1970s. Next came condoms and birth control pills. They accounted for 42.5%, 24.3%, and 19.4% of birth control efforts, respectively.[66]

Fallopian tube surgery was performed beginning in the early 1970s. The loop and the oral contraceptive pill had seemed economical, but the dropout rate and discontinuation rate were high enough to make them inefficient and ineffective. In contrast, the operation was irreversible, and its contraceptive effect was high. Therefore, since the 1970s, there has been a strong argument that "the priority should be given to recommending surgery."[67] In the 1980s, the rate of vasectomies began to rise. The ratio of vasectomies increased to one fourth of fallopian tube surgery in 1982, one third in 1983, and one half in 1984.

This was because there were several benefits, including a winning ticket for an apartment and early release from reserve forces training.[68] Moreover, the men who participated in the project had families with an average size of four children, including, on average, more than two sons. In a sense, they had already achieved what they had hoped for.[69] In 1992, the ratio of male to female sterilization was 54.9:54.1, which means that for the first time since the implementation of the family planning project, the proportion of sterilized men exceeded that of women.[70]

The national average of 5.8 children in 1961 decreased to 2.6 in 1979. It had halved in 20 years.[71] The family planning project succeeded in suppressing population growth. Support from foreign institutions was yet again one of the most important success factors. Among them, the support of the American PathFinder Fund and the American Population Council was important.[72]

However, the most important success factor was active cooperation between the government and the people. Only the Catholic Church opposed the project, as the government allowed abortion to control the population. Even Protestants participated in the family planning project.[73] It is hardly possible to find resistance from mothers against the family planning project. Older generations—particularly elderly males in rural areas—showed an aversion to the project, but due to the extensive publicity and change in society, the aversion disappeared by the 1970s.[74]

At the center of the integration of the government and the people was Korean society's goal of economic growth. The government regarded the family planning project as another economic development plan and promoted it accordingly. Citizens also joined. Family planning was an opportunity for parents who dreamed of entering a higher class to obtain a better education for their children.[75] The family planning project was "a part of the economic development policy, a welfare policy for living well together."[76] Economic growth and development was the force that unified Korean society in the 1960s and 1970s.

The Implementation of a Medical Insurance System and Increasing Medical Demand

The number of doctors of Western medicine had steadily increased during the colonial period, from 641 in 1914 to 3,674 in 1942. This increase gave people more opportunities to see medical doctors. However, as medical fees were not cheap and most medical doctors worked in cities, seeing medical doctors was hardly possible for many, particularly people in rural areas.

Medical insurance could solve this problem to a certain degree. In 1938, health insurance arose in Japan to ensure that members belonging to the National Health Insurance Association were entitled to free treatment in case of illness.[77] After the introduction of health insurance in Japan, there were calls for the same system in colonial Korea. However, implementing this system required a significant budget.[78] If the budget problem was not resolved, laws related to health insurance could not be implemented.

Medical insurance was legally introduced in 1963. It was intended to provide insurance benefits in the event of illness, injury, death, or childbirth to workers or dependents in the same situations for reasons other than work. People in rural areas and nonindustrial workers were not involved in this system. According to this act, employers who regularly employed 300 or more workers could establish a medical insurance union with the consent of 300 or more workers and approval from the Minister of Public Health and Social

Affairs. This meant that the system was legally launched. At least superficially, the military government felt the need for a social security act like medical insurance that covered the entire nation. However, it had no practical meaning because a system of voluntary enrollment in medical institutions was adopted. The medical institution that signed the contract could, at any time, ask the minister of public health and social affairs to cancel the contract. The contract between the insurer and the medical institution was thus not only voluntary but also loose.[79]

It was difficult to settle for medical insurance that consisted of voluntary enrollment. Insurance finances deteriorated as subjects with high medical use rates signed up for insurance, and in many cases, the insured could not receive benefits due to the limitations on medical treatments. "In the end, mandatory medical insurance would be the only solution."[80]

In the 1970s, the situation did not improve significantly. The problem of the financial resources required for the insurance business had not yet been resolved. The business community was against medical insurance. The Federation of Korean Industries argued, for example, that "it is still too early for Korea, which is not a developed country, to implement medical insurance."[81] Concerns about the financial burden were also shared by the private sector. An individual who established and operated a health cooperative argued that such a business was a realistic way to "expand the pilot project of health cooperatives as much as possible" until the national income increased.[82]

However, it is said that President Park Chung-hee had a strong policy drive to implement medical insurance. His determination needs to be understood against the background that inequality and rifts in society began to appear as the economic development plan paid off. The 1970s witnessed the side effects of economic growth, such as overurbanization and standard-of-living discrepancies. The Fourth Republic began with the promulgation of the Yushin Constitution in 1972, which stipulated a highly powerful authoritarian system; in response, the opposition increased its demands for a broadening of human rights and an amelioration of the plight of labor.[83] The government needed to calm the dissatisfaction in society caused by economic development. Medical insurance could be such a balm.

The government's will to implement medical insurance was declared in March 1976 through the "Measures to Expand Medical Benefits to Improve National Health." In this announcement, the government made it clear that by establishing a basis for national health care, they would institutionalize measures to disperse and reduce the burden of medical expenses through medical insurance for the public.[84]

In July 1977, the medical insurance system was implemented. It copied the Japanese system in three respects: the administrative structure of the system, the choice about who would be covered, and the policy for mobilizing financial resources for the system. Although American medicine had a dominant influence on the development of Korean medicine, the American model was not fit for South Korea because the United States had failed to achieve a compulsory, universal medical insurance system.[85]

When the medical insurance system was first launched, it was applied to workplaces with 500 or more workers and workers in industrial complexes. It was difficult to expand the scope of compulsory application to all workers at once because not all employers and employees could afford a certain amount of medical insurance fees. Employees were expected to earn enough to pay half the premium. At that time, the coverage range was 498 unions, about 1.1 million insured persons, and about 1.9 million dependents—thus, about 3 million people in total, accounting for 8.2% of the total population. When the 2.1 million people in medical care were integrated, it equaled 14% of the total population.

As the demand for expanding insurance coverage increased, the sizes of the workplaces covered by medical insurance gradually shrank. In 1982, workplaces with 16 or more employees were included, and workplaces with five or more employees could also be covered, if desired. In 1981, medical insurance was extended to residents living in rural areas.[86] The nature of regional medical insurance changed from voluntary to compulsory.[87] The scope of compulsory application was to be expanded in stages.

The fee paid to medical personnel was decided on a fee-for-service basis, in accordance with the opinions of doctors. Among the proposed systems, the fee-for-service system was most similar to the existing service system. There was no alternative other than fee for service to forcefully designate the price and payment compensation for medical services, which were freely determined under the market economy system.[88]

The doctors were not satisfied. The government claimed that the fee provided by medical insurance reached about 75% of the conventional fee. Furthermore, they persuaded doctors that insurance would not only guarantee medical expenses but also increase medical demand.[89] The Medical Association issued a correction, pointing out that the determined fee was only 55% of the conventional fee. They added that medical insurance would deprive sick people of the right to choose medical institutions and, conversely, encourage the trend of medical shopping. Medical insurance was also accused of creating competition, such as expansions of facilities by rival medical doctors. The Medical Association used the media to publicize these medical insurance issues.[90]

The medical insurance system in South Korea was established at the expense of Korean doctors' incomes and autonomy. Doctors, however, had no choice but to passively condone the launch of medical insurance.[91] It would have been difficult for the medical community to reject the system the government wanted to implement under the Yushin system, in which all power was concentrated in the president. This was a time when one could get caught and dragged away to nowhere for making a dissenting statement in public against government policies. Doctors had to endure and follow orders from above.[92] To cope, they temporarily compensated for the deficits caused by medical insurance with the income of uninsured patients.[93] They used other expedients as well. Drug price margins were one of the main ways to make up the losses: "Medical institutions had no choice but to cover losses from medical insurance treatment with profits from drug prices and non-coverage."[94]

According to a survey conducted in 1978, with the introduction of medical insurance, patients' preference for general hospitals increased. According to a report written in the 1950s, the confidence of the public in private practitioners was higher than that in hospital doctors.[95] The bed occupancy rate of general hospitals, which was 39.1% before the implementation of medical insurance, increased to 41.7% in less than a year. Conversely, the bed occupancy rate of private practitioners decreased from 32.9% to 28.6%.[96] Another survey showed that 12.3% of the clinics designated as medical insurance institutions did not treat even one insured patient for 11 months after the insurance program was implemented.[97] It is clear that medical insurance strengthened patients' preference for general hospitals.

Now that medical insurance had emerged, the need to expand it increased. In the early 1980s, the difference between the medical insurance fee and the general fee was 100:157—a difference of more than 1.5 times. It was natural for those who did not have medical insurance to demand that insurance coverage be expanded.[98] To cover all regions, the government subsidized 50% of the total financial requirement. It was at the same level as the support that employees received from their employers. The 50% support of insurance finance was unprecedented in the world,[99] the support decreased every year, however. In 1989, medical insurance expanded to cover all South Korean people. Within 12 years, South Korea went from private, voluntary medical insurance to universal, government-mandated coverage.

The Weakening of Public Medicine and Growth of Private Hospitals

In colonial Korea, a private medical system was in effect. Provincial hospitals were established in provincial areas by the colonial government, and poor patients—in particular, Korean patients—were treated free of charge, at least in the first stage of colonial rule. However, as the 1920s passed, provincial hospitals began to operate primarily for medical treatment profits. A private practice system of physicians was also established. In medieval Korea, doctors called *Yu-ui* (Confucius doctors) performed the benevolent act of providing free medical care to the residents of the areas in which they lived. As the commercialization of medical care progressed during the colonial period, some doctors suggested a shift away from this benevolent art. In the colonial period, the pursuit of profit through medical practice began to be taken for granted.[100]

At the same time, voices calling for state intervention or management in medicine also spread. The adoption of socialist ideas in the 1920s was an important moment in this respect. After liberation, the left oriented itself toward the nationalization of medical care as the ultimate goal. Although the system of private practice was maintained, the left intended to gradually promote the socialization of medical care. Specifically, they aimed to reduce the proportion of private practitioners through the expansion of state-run hospitals.[101]

As the left–right conflict over the liberation space ended in the victory for the right, a private medical system was established in South Korea. This system was instrumental for Cold War ideological propaganda, as it emphasized the superiority of the American ideals of democracy and liberalism. The private practice-centered system continued to exacerbate two well-known problems during the colonial period—the urban concentration of doctors and the concomitant increase in the number of doctorless villages.[102]

The social situation after the Korean War also made it difficult for the government to make public investments in medical care. As a result, the share of the public sector in medical care decreased with the private sector's growth. In 1959 alone, the number of beds in national and public hospitals accounted for 67% of the total number of beds. However, the proportion gradually decreased—to 48% in 1966, 41% in 1973, and 31% in 1980.

Medical insurance, launched in 1977, rapidly increased the demand for medical care, and private hospitals were the beneficiaries. As of 1980, the proportion of medical personnel working in city and municipal hospitals was only 0.01% of all doctors and 0.01% of nurses, including nursing assistants. The national and public hospitals were not able to fulfill their role as modern medical institutions due to the outdated facilities and equipment.[103] The share of the public sector in medical supply was clearly shrinking. It was also clear that medical support for vulnerable social groups would be reduced.

The private sector also encouraged measures to increase medical manpower. Beginning in the mid-1970s, 15 medical schools were newly established over 10 years; as a result, the number of medical schools increased from 14 in 1975 to 29 in 1987. It is noteworthy that only two of these universities were national.[104] Private medical schools were active in the establishment and expansion of hospitals and began to establish themselves as the center of the medical system. An example is the *chaebol* hospitals (conglomerate hospitals) established from the late 1980s to the early 1990s.

The government also relied on the private sector to provide medical care to marginalized areas. Loans lent by Japan and domestic banks were provided for the establishment of private medical facilities.[105] However, hospitals established in marginalized areas were prone to insufficient medical demand, difficulties in securing medical personnel, inexperienced hospital management, and financial difficulties in the early stages of opening. The result was, in severe cases, bankruptcy. Even in such cases, the government tried to solve these problems by relying on the private sector. A large-scale hospital with extensive experience in hospital operation and sound financial capabilities was asked to take over the bankrupt hospitals.[106] In the 1980s, the government's policy to solve medical problems in medically marginalized areas continued, primarily through the establishment of private rather than public hospitals.

Private hospitals could fill the void in the medical supply when the state's financial or operational capacities were insufficient. The private-centered medical system contributed to meeting the public's medical demand without a heavy budgetary burden during the economic growth period when available resources were scarce.[107] Public health centers also continued to serve as primary medical institutions focusing on patient care, particularly in rural areas. As the local self-government system was implemented, the focus was also placed on managing the health of local residents.

The problem was that there was no comprehensive plan at the government level regarding the support and utilization of the private sector. The government did not have a strategy for or approach to developing the private sector. As the financial role of the government in the operation of the medical system had been minor, it had no means to effectively control the private sector.[108] The private-centered medical system, which was launched after liberation in South Korea, has been strengthened through the period of economic growth.

Conclusion

During the period of economic growth from the 1960s through the 1980s, the medical system in South Korea grew and became systematized. The government agency responsible for public health was clarified, and several laws related to medical care were passed. Nationwide anti-epidemic projects were initiated, and several infectious diseases were reduced. The period of economic growth was also, therefore, the period in which the origins of Korea's present medical system were established.

Public health centers were at the center of anti-epidemic disease activities and family planning, although they were criticized for putting more effort into medical treatment than public health. While private hospitals began to play a major role in the medical supply, public health centers represented public concerns in South Korea. In 1966, prevention laws on tuberculosis and parasite control were enacted. Based on these laws, the Korean Tuberculosis Association conducted a nationwide survey on tuberculosis infection, and the Korea Association of Eradication of Parasites conducted a survey on parasite infection. They played a pivotal role by suggesting related project proposals to the government and academically supporting them through research.

The role of the Korean people was also crucial. Without the participation of the Korean people in the anti-epidemic projects, such large-scale efforts could never have materialized. Students had to submit smelly stool envelopes to school and take parasiticide with all eyes on them if they got a positive result. People in rural areas used to stand in front of X-ray machines to check whether they had contracted tuberculosis. It is not easy to find signs of resistance or rejection among Koreans in this era.

Above all, the medical insurance system was founded in South Korea in 1977. It was only able to cover the employees of large companies, at least in the first stage. However, the establishment of medical insurance meant that Korea finally had a reliable social safety net in the public health field. Without the determination of the Korean government, suppressing the objection of medical doctors and launching the medical insurance system would have been unthinkable.

The 1960s was the time to restart the effort to establish a postcolonial modern state. The military government was keen on developing public health programs to shore up their legitimacy. It argued that fostering people's health was a good way to secure a healthy workforce, thereby advancing South Korea's priorities in economic development. The Korean people were willing to participate in the project to economically grow their country. As they experienced a series of trials—from liberation to civil war within a span of less than a decade—securing a safe and developed country was a natural desire. In the public health field, anti-epidemic programs were efforts in which the Korean people would participate. Just after the liberation of Korea in 1945, the illiteracy rate was about 78%. However, thanks to the dissemination of primary education and a campaign to abolish illiteracy, the rate was reduced to 8.8% in 1966 and 7% in 1970. They were a highly literate population with a willingness to embrace change.

However, it would be a mistake to approach the development of the public health sector in South Korea only from a domestic viewpoint. Foreign aid—for instance, from the WHO, UNICEF, or the OTCA—inaugurated anti-epidemic projects. The WHO and UNICEF provided technical and financial support for a nationwide tuberculosis survey, and the anti-parasite program took root with the help of Japan's OTCA. In the case of family planning, U.S. population organizations played the same role as other international agencies.

The Cold War was the ideological basis for this international support. Family planning was conceived to prevent developing, mired in poverty, from being communist countries. As Japan was assigned to support liberal countries in East Asia, it promoted anti-parasite activities in South Korea through the OTCA. In the 1960s, Korea had a strong authoritarian government that was able to utilize international support. Things had changed since the 1940s and 1950s when the newborn government could not exercise its leadership except by inspiring anti-communist sentiments.

However, the Korean government has focused only on the dimensions of public health directly related to the growth of the economy. Family planning is a typical example. It was driven only by a means of coping with the population problem, and there was no comprehensive vision. Parasite eradication programs and anti-tuberculosis activities proceeded, as they could cultivate healthy citizens as a robust labor force. However, the Korean government paid little attention to projects that demanded financial investment and long-term planning. Public health projects were promoted for economic development and growth.

As a result, the Korean government's main achievement in the public health domain was its anti-epidemic activities. As public hospitals served increasingly fewer patients, private hospitals began to play a larger role in the medical supply. The medical insurance system, to be sure, owed its launch to government

initiatives. However, after the emergence of this system, the role the government assumed was medicating the insurer and the insured, not assuming a
financial burden. Anything that did not directly promote economic growth
could not be a concern for the Korean government. It showed little interest in
investing in the public health sector any further. It is no surprise, then, that the
private medical sector in South Korea continues to gradually expand. When
discussing the current state of medical care in South Korea, securing publicity
promises to be an increasingly important issue.

Notes

1 John Dimoia, *Reconstructing Bodies: Biomedicine, Health, and Nation-Building in South Korea Since 1945* (Stanford: Stanford University Press, 2013).
2 Ibid., 6.
3 Shin Dong-won, "Public Health and People's Health: Contrasting the Paths of Healthcare Systems in South and North Korea, 1945–60," in *Public Health and National Reconstruction in Post-War Asia*, eds. Liping Bu and Ka-che Yip (London and New York: Routledge, 2014), 100–103.
4 Jane Sung Hae Kim, "Securitizing Health: Biosecurity and Postwar Reconstruction in Korea," *The Korean Journal for the History of Science* 44, no. 2 (2022): 284–286.
5 *Bogeonsahoihaengjeonggaegwan* [Health and Social Administration Overview], (Seoul: Ministry of Public Health and Society, 1958), 170.
6 WHO/UNKRA, Report of the Health Planning Mission in Korea, Feb. 26, (1953): 30–34.
7 *Bogeonsahoibaekseo 1964* [public health white paper 1964], (Seoul: Ministry of Public Health and Society, 1965), 52–53.
8 *Bogeonsahoi 1982* [Public Health and Society 1982], (Seoul: Ministry of Public Health and Society, 1982), 149.
9 *Bogeonsahoi 1987* [Public Health and Society 1987], (Seoul: Ministry of Public Health and Society, 1987), 70.
10 *Bogeonjubo* [Public Health Weekly Report], Oct. 13, (1995): 9
11 Daehanbogeonhyeophoi, *Daehanminguk Bogeonbaldalsa* [A History of Public Health in Korea], (Seoul: Daehanbogeonhyeophoi, 2014), 78.
12 *Bogeonsahoi 1981* [Public Health and Society 1981], (Seoul: Ministry of Public Health and Society, 1981), 56.
13 Ibid., 49.
14 *Bogeonsahoibaekseo 1964*, 67.
15 Kim Kyuri et al., "Infrastructure-building for Public Health: The World Health Organization and Tuberculosis Control in South Korea, 1945–1963", *Uisahak* [Korean Journal of Medical History] 28, no. 1 (2019): 92.
16 *Bogeonsahoi 1981*, 59–60.
17 *Bogeonsahoibaekseo 1964*, 67.
18 The Korean Tuberculosis Association, *Daehangyeolhaekhyeophoi 20nyeonsa* [20-year history of the Korean Tuberculosis Association], (Seoul, The Korean Tuberculosis Association, 1974), 130.
19 The Korean Tuberculosis Association, *Daehangyeolhaekhyeophoi 30nyeonsa* [30-year history of the Korean Tuberculosis Association], (Seoul, The Korean Tuberculosis Association, 1983), 209.
20 Kim Kyuri et al., Infrastructure-building for Public Health, 114–115.
21 The Korean Tuberculosis Association, *Daehangyeolhaekhyeophoi 20nyeonsa*, 95, 98.

22 The Law on Tuberculosis Prevention, enacted Jan. 16 (1967).
23 Sherwood Hall, *With Stethoscope in Asia: Korea* (Mclean, MCL ASSOCIATE, 1978), 418–420, 443.
24 *Bogeonsahoi 1981*, 49.
25 Ibid., 102.
26 *Bogeonsahoibaekseo 1964*, 67.
27 Daehanminguk Haksulwon, *Hangukeu Haksulyeongu* [Academic Research of Korea], (Seoul: Daehanminguk Haksulwon, 2004), 50.
28 *Jungangbangyeokyeonguso Sobo* [Report of Central Quarantine Research Institute] 1, no. 1 (1949): 49.
29 The Korea Association of Health Promotion, *Geonhyeop40nyeonsa* [40-year History of Korea Association of Health Promotion], (Seoul: The Korea Association of Health Promotion, 2005), 104–105.
30 Soh Chin-Thack, "Parasitic Diseases in Rural Area of Korea and the Control," (in Korean) *Journal of Korean Medical Association* 9, no. 6 (1966): 26.
31 Parasitic Disease Prevention Act enacted Apr. 25 (1966).
32 The Korea Association of Health Promotion, *Geonhyeop40nyeonsa*. 109.
33 Lee Soon-hyung, "Geogukgeok Gisangchung Jipdangwanri Saeopui Chuji" [Promotion of national parasite group management project], *Hanguk Gisangchunggyamyeomui Yeongu Mit Toechi* [Research and eradication of parasitic infections in Korea], (Seoul: Daehanmingukhaksulwon, 2007): 133.
34 The Korea Association on Eradication of Parasites, *Gihyeopisimnyeonsa* [20-year History of Korea Association on Eradication of Parasites], (Seoul: The Korea Association on Eradication of Parasites, 1984), 105.
35 The Korea Association of Health Promotion, *Geohyeopisasimnyeonsa*, 113.
36 Byong Seol Seo, "On the Present Status and Prospect of the Parasite Control Problems in Korea" (in Korean), *Journal of Korean Medical Association* 22, no. 11, (1979): 902.
37 The Korea Association on Eradication of Parasites, *Gihyeopisimnyeonsa*, 107.
38 The Korea Association of Health Promotion, *Geohyeopisasimnyeonsa*, 112.
39 Daehanminguk Haksulwon, *Hangukeu Haksulyeongu*, 239.
40 Lee Soon-hyung, "Geogukgeok Gisangchung Jipdangwanri Saeopui Chuji," 175–179.
41 Ibid., 182.
42 The Korea Association on Eradication of Parasites, *Gihyeopisimnyeonsa*, 51.
43 Ibid., 49.
44 The Korea Association on Eradication of Parasites, *Hanguk Haksaeng Hoichunggamyeom Jipdangwanrisaeop Bunseok* [Analysis of group management project for roundworm infection of Korean students], (Seoul, The Korea Association on Eradication of Parasites, 1980), 5.
45 John Dimoia, *Reconstructing Bodies*, 175.
46 Junho Jung et al., "A Social History of Ascariasis in the 1960s Korea: From a Norm to a Shameful Disease," (in Korean) *Korean Journal of Medical History* 25, no. 2 (2016): 187.
47 The Korea Association on Eradication of Parasites, *Gihyeopisimnyeonsa*, 51.
48 Bogeonbokji70nyeonsapyeonchanuiwonhoi, *Bogeonbokji70nyeonsa* [70-year History of Public Health and Welfare], (Sejong: Ministry of Public Health and Welfare, 2015): 293.
49 Bae Eun-Kyung, *Hyeondae Hangukui Ingan Jaesaengsan* [Human reproduction in modern Korea], (Seoul: Siganyeohaeng, 2012): 87–92.
50 Korea Association of Family Planning, *Hangukgajokgyeohoiksimnyeonsa* [10-year history of Korean family planning], (Seoul: Korea Association of Family Planning, 1975): 29, 193–194.

51 In-Sok Yeo, "A history of public health in Korea," *Public health in Asia and the Pacific* (London: Routledge, 2008), 83.
52 Kim Yong Wan, "Family Planning Program in Korea", (in Korean) *Journal of Korean Medical Association* 7, no. 6 (1964): 518.
53 John Dimoia, *Reconstructing Bodies*, 114–117.
54 Bogeonbokji70nyeonsapyeonchanuiwonhoi, *Bogeonbokji70nyeonsa*, 298.
55 Korea Association of Family Planning, *Hangukgajokgyeohoiksimnyeonsa*, 69.
56 John Dimoia, *Reconstructing Bodies*, 118–119.
57 Kim Myung Ho, "Health Activities in Rural Korea" (in Korean), *Journal of Korean Medical Association* 9, no. 6 (1966): 38–40.
58 Bogeonsahoibaekseo 1991 [public health white paper 1991], (Seoul: Ministry of Public Health and Society, 1991): 8–9.
59 Ibid., 268.
60 *Bogeonsahoi 1981*, 269.
61 Maternal and Child Health Act enacted Feb. 8 (1973).
62 Korea Association of Family Planning, *Hangukgajokgyeohoiksimnyeonsa*, 102.
63 *Bogeonsahoi 1981*, 26–70.
64 Shin Han Su et al., "Intra-uterine Device," (in Korean), *Journal of Korean Medical Association* 13, no. 5 (1970): 398.
65 John Dimoia, *Reconstructing Bodies*, p. 123.
66 *Bogeonsahoi 1981*, 270.
67 Korea Association of Family Planning, *Hangukgajokgyeohoiksimnyeonsa*, 43
68 *Gyeonghyang Sinmun* [Gyeonghyang Newspaper], Sep. 8, (1977).
69 John Dimoia, *Reconstructing Bodies*, 133.
70 *Bogeonsahoi 1993* [Public Health and Society 1993], (Seoul: Ministry of Public Health and Society, 1993), 74.
71 *Bogeonsahoi 1981*, 275.
72 Yang Jae-Mo, *Sarangui Bichman Jigo* [I owe a lot to others] (Seoul: Qline, 2001), 308.
73 Kang In-Chul, *Jeohanggwa Tuhang* [Resistance and Surrender], (Osan: Hanshin University Press, 2013), 366–367, 402.
74 Bae Eun-Kyung, *Hyeondae Hangukui Ingan Jaesaengsan*, 114.
75 Ibid., 199–206.
76 Yang Jae-Mo, *Sarangui Bichman Jigo*, 373–375.
77 *Chosun Ilbo* [Chosun Daily News] May 25, (1938).
78 *Chosun Ilbo* [Chosun Daily News] May 4, (1939).
79 *Bogeonsahoi 1981*, 176.
80 Medical Insurance Association, *Uiryoboheomui Baljachui* [The footsteps of Medical insurance], (Seoul: Medical Insurance Association, 1997), 70–71.
81 Ibid., 87.
82 Chang Kee Ryo, "On Medical Insurance in Korea" (in Korean), *Journal of Korean Medical Association* 15, no. 11 (1972): 894.
83 Michael E. Robinson, *Korea's Twentieth-Century Odyssey* (Honolulu: University of Hawaii Press, 2007), 137.
84 Medical Insurance Association, *Uiryoboheomui Baljachui*, 83.
85 Jong-Chan Lee, "Health Care Reform in South Korea – Success or Failure," *American Journal of Public Health* 93, no. 1 (2003): 48–49.
86 Medical Insurance Act partly revised Apr. 4, (1981).
87 Bogeonbokji70nyeonsapyeonchanuiwonhoi, *Bogeonbokji70nyeonsa*, 376.
88 Bogeonbokji70nyeonsapyeonchanuiwonhoi, *Bogeonbokji70nyeonsa*, 412.
89 "About Korea's medical insurance system" (in Korean), *Journal of Korean Medical Association* 20, no. 6 (1977): 553.
90 Seoul Medical Association, *Seoulteukbyeolsieuisahoi 100nyeonsa* [The 100th Anniversary Seoul Medical Association], (Seoul: Seoul Medical Association, 2016), 154–155.

91 Medical Insurance Association, *Uiryoboheomui Baljachui*, 143.
92 Eungeong Ma, *Medicine in the Making in Post-colonial Korea (1948–2006)*, (PhD. diss., Cornell University, 2008): 118–119.
93 Myung Do Song, "Korean National Medical Insurance System Compared with Other Nations," (in Korean), *Journal of Korean Medical Association* 25, no. 1 (1982): 21.
94 Han Joong Kim, "Expansion of medical insurance finances and reasonable adjustment of medical fees," (in Korean) *Journal of Korean Medical Association* 43, no. 10 (2000): 980.
95 WHO/UNKRA, Report of the Health Planning Mission in Korea, Feb. 26, (1953): 5.
96 Medical Insurance Association, *Uiryoboheomui Baljachui*, 145.
97 Youngbo Sim, "The First Year Experience of Health Insurance in Korea" (in Korean), *Journal of Korean Medical Association* 21, no. 9 (1978): 736–737.
98 *Bogeonsahoi 1982*, 250.
99 *Bogeonsahoi 1990* [Public Health and Society 1990], (Seoul: Ministry of Public Health and Society, 1990): 5.
100 Park Yunjae, "Commercialization of Medicine in the Late 19th and Early 20th Century in Korea," *Korea Journal* 55, no. 2 (2015): 49–55.
101 Choi Uing Seok, "Fundamental duties of health administration at the present stage" (in Korean), Joseonuihaksinbo [Korean Medical News] 2 (1947): 19.
102 Shin Dong-won, "Public Health and People's Health," 100–103.
103 *Bogeonsahoi 1981*, 87.
104 The Korea Public Health Association, *Daehanminguk Bogeonbaldalsa* [The History of Public Health Development in South Korea], (Seoul: The Korea Public Health Association, 2014), 36–37.
105 *Bogeonsahoi 1984* [Public Health and Society 1984], (Seoul: Ministry of Public Health and Society, 1984), 211.
106 *Bogeonsahoi 1986* [Public Health and Society 1986], (Seoul: Ministry of Public Health and Society, 1986), 211.
107 Bogeonbokjibaekseo 2006 [Public Health and Welfare White Paper 2006), (Seoul: Ministry of Public Health and welfare, 2006), 422.
108 The Korea Public Health Association, *Daehanminguk Bogeonbaldalsa*, 34, 37.

4 Health Insurance Policy and Its Stakeholders in Japan during the Cold War

Toward the Introduction of Universal Health Care*

Takakazu Yamagishi

Introduction

The Cold War affected the health insurance politics and policies in Japan but probably in a more complicated way than in other Asian countries. When the Cold War began, Japan was under US-led occupation. The General Headquarters of the Supreme Commander for the Allied Powers (SCAP/GHQ) had supreme power in making new health insurance policies. Moreover, by the end of the war, Japan had developed a quasi-universal health care system. The first major health insurance policy was the Health Insurance Act of 1922 that targeted manual workers. Additionally, the government's war mobilization policy resulted in the coverage expansion of national health insurance programs, including the establishment of the National Health Insurance Act of 1938. The effect of the Cold War needs to be examined in these historical and institutional contexts.

This chapter demonstrates how the Cold War affected health insurance policies up to the introduction of universal health care in 1961 by paying special attention to medical associations and labor organizations in the existing institutional and political environment. Hence, this chapter begins with an overview of the health insurance system that was in place in 1961. Subsequently, it explains how health insurance policies developed in the political context that was created before the war ended. It moves on to discuss how the Cold War influenced the health insurance politics and policies during the US-led occupation. This chapter concludes by examining how the Cold War influenced the movement to create the universal health insurance system in 1961.

The Health Insurance System in 1961

When Japan achieved universal health care in 1961, the health insurance system was composed of multiple programs that targeted different groups depending on their employment status. Each program had a different insurer, premium, and copayment; but they shared the same national health insurance

* The research was supported by JSPS KAKENHI Grant Number 22K01345 and the Pache Research Subsidy I-A-2 for Academic Year 2023 of Nanzan University.

DOI: 10.4324/9781003318163-5

fee system. This system affected how political actors, including medical professionals and laborers, acted to approach the policymaking process.[1]

Those who worked in big companies joined the Society-Managed Health Insurance (SMHI). Companies with more than 500 workers were mandated to set up and run their own mutual society for their employees. Those who worked in smaller companies joined the Government-Managed Health Insurance (GMHI). The government was the sole insurer of the program. These two programs were established by the Health Insurance Act of 1922 (HI).[2]

If one is self-employed, as in the case of farmers and fishermen, the person is required to join the National Health Insurance program run by the municipality they reside in. All municipalities were required to create and administer their programs. Within the national government's regulation, each municipality decided the premium depending on its financial condition. The age and financial averages of the enrollees of the NHI were poorer than the HI because the retirees, the aged, participated in the NHI. As a result, the NHI programs were usually inferior to the HI, especially in terms of premium and copayment. The NHI enrollees paid about a 50 percent copayment while the HI enrollees paid a minimum copayment.

What gave this fragmented administration uniformity was the common national health insurance fee system. The Central Social Insurance Medical Council (Shakaihoken Iryō Kyōgikai, called Chūikyō) decided the fees for medical services and prescription drugs. The council included medical service providers (doctors), insurers, employers, the insured, and policy experts. Whenever new medical technologies and medicine were to be included in national health insurance coverage, the government was required to have reports of the council.[3]

Japan introduced this universal health insurance system in 1961, but it took many decades to develop the government's intervention in health care finance and create public health insurance programs. The problems for Japan were that the government faced international pressures to modernize and strengthen the country. Health insurance policy became a tool for the government to do so. Hence, the health insurance system in Japan was built in haste rather than a deliberate approach of debate and discussion.

Built in Haste

Japan ended the feudal Tokugawa regime in 1868 when the Tokugawa shogunate decided to return the governing authority to the emperor. The external pressures, including Commodore Matthew Perry's visit to Japan with black ships, triggered the power transformation. However, by providing unequal treaties such as giving up extraterritorial rights and tariff autonomy to major Western nations, Japan continued to be under pressure to modernize and strengthen the nation.

The newly established Meiji government pushed hard for its Westernization project eventually to demolish the unequal treaties and expand its power in the international community to join Western imperial powers. Expanding the military and developing industries were priorities for the government. Health policy became part of the government's Westernization project as a means, first, to deal with epidemics and control the public order and, second, to improve workers' health levels and economic productivity. Health insurance mainly dealt with the second part of the project.

The bad working conditions made young workers sick and injured. It not only lowered the productivity of companies but also caused social anxiety. Labor movements meantime began to spread. Many bureaucrats, including Shinpei Gotō,[4] studied in Europe to see how the governments there dealt with such problems.

The establishment of the HI in 1922 resulted from these bureaucrats' research. It included the SMHI for employees of large companies and the GMHI for employees of smaller companies. The government used the existing scheme to create the SMHI. Many large companies had already established their own mutual associations to provide health insurance, medical, and other services for their workers. The HI incorporated them with the government's regulations as the SMHI. On the other hand, because the GMHI was established from scratch, the government gained legitimacy to become the sole insurer of the program. As a result, the government played a role both in supervising the entire HI and in administering the GMHI.[5]

The creation of the HI resulted largely from party politics in post–World War I Japan. As universal male suffrage was approaching, the Kenseikai Party and the Seiyūkai Party used the HI to appeal to the people in urban areas. Without revisions, the bill was passed with "surprising speed."[6] It was top-down legislation with no serious efforts to compromise with stakeholders. Moreover, the number of HI enrollees did not increase much after its establishment.[7]

While the GMHI targeted employees in smaller companies, the program did not include ones in micro enterprises with fewer than 10 employees. Additionally, farmers, still a predominant workforce, were left out of the HI. The HI was also unpopular among doctors. Doctors had a tradition of self-pay practice. Many doctors refused to take patients with the HI. This deadlock situation changed because military action abroad pressured the government to invest more in health care.

The Mukden Incident of 1931 isolated Japan in the international community and prepared it for future large-scale wars. The health of young men, particularly in rural areas, became important for the army as this was the source for enrolling soldiers. Farmers suffered from the Great Depression, and many did not have access to medical services. As described, the HI did not reach farmers at that time. For its political purpose, the army urged the government to create a new ministry in the area of public health and introduce a new national health insurance program for farmers.

As the war in China became longer and more devastating in the 1930s than anticipated, the government concluded that the health of the people became crucial to national security. The government needed healthy soldiers and workers to win the war. It had to avoid inefficacies in war mobilization; it had to reduce the number of young men who failed the physical examination for conscription and workers who were absent due to injuries and sickness. The more intense the war became, the harder the government pushed for the expansion of health insurance.[8]

After the Ministry of Health and Welfare was established in 1938, the NHI was the first legislation for the new ministry. The NHI was established as a voluntary program. NHI mutual associations were to be set up, and municipalities were to supervise them. Because the enrollees were mostly farmers, unlike the HI, there were no employers who contributed part of the premium. The government paid the administrative cost, but that was obviously not enough. The number of NHI enrollees did not increase as much as the government desired because there was no strong incentive for people to voluntarily form the NHI mutual associations.

The NHI appeared to be a major achievement in the development of health insurance, but it symbolizes that the health insurance system was still like a paper tiger, looking good but possessing no sufficient substance. With the wartime necessity to mobilize many young people to win the war, the government had a justification for expanding the paper-tiger health insurance system as cheaply as possible.

As the war continued, the government sought to improve the health insurance system, but it did not have much financial leeway to invest in health care because of the increase in war expenses. The health insurance system with the new NHI remained a paper tiger. Private stakeholders, such as laborers and medical professionals, did not show much influence in the policymaking process to improve the policy substance because they were enmeshed in the government's war activities.

Labor unions had been generally seen by the government as a disturbance to public order. When the Meiji government advanced its industrialization policy, it largely neglected the issue of working conditions for workers. As the labor movement emerged in the late nineteenth century, the government, in response, issued the Public Order and Police Provisions Act (Chian Keisatsu Hō) that allowed the Ministry of Home (Naimu Shō) and the policy to gain strong control over labor movement and damage their assemblies.[9] Later, more moderate labor unions were created,[10] but they did not gain formal powers such as the right to collectively bargain with employers.

As the war intensified in the 1930s, the political parties and the labor unions lost their autonomy. In 1938, the National Mobilization Act (Kokka Sōdōin Hō) was established. In 1940, all political parties were dissolved to join a new state organization, the Imperial Rule Assistance Association (Taisei Yokusankai). Labor unions were also dismissed and forced to join the Industrial Association for Serving the Nation (Sangyō Hōkokukai). Labor unions completely became the arm of the government to pursue the war goals.

Like labor unions, medical professionals also lost their autonomy during the war. However, the beginning of medical associations was different from that of labor unions. As noted, the Meiji government's Westernization policy included the Westernization of medicine. The internal wars proved that traditional medicine, the Japanese adoption of Chinese medicine, did not serve well for surgeries. The government decided to completely change Japanese medicine into Western medicine by creating a hierarchical medical education system topped by Tokyo Imperial University.[11]

As more doctors practiced Western medicine, medical associations emerged. However, doctors of Western medicine benefited from the government's policy on medicine, and therefore, their main political enemy was initially not the government but doctors of traditional Japanese medicine. Both sides sought to mobilize fellow doctors to pressure the government. The political battle ended with the victory of Western-style doctors.[12] In the early twentieth century when the government began to be involved in health insurance, Western-style doctors increasingly saw the government as an obstacle to their financial interest. But their relationship remained less than completely adversarial until the mid-1930s.

The government had a different interest in doctors from labor unions. Japan did not have extensively developed public hospitals. The deflationary policy in the 1880s, led by Finance Minister Masayoshi Matsukata, had a large impact on this trend. It did not allow prefectures to use local tax revenues for public medical schools. As a result, many public hospitals attached to the medical schools were sold to the private sector.[13] The government had to adopt a more careful attitude toward doctors than labor unions because the Japanese health care system relied chiefly on private hospitals, clinics, and doctors.

When the HI of 1922 was discussed, the government consulted with elite private doctors in the Greater Japan Medical Association (GJMA), then a national yet voluntary association. The government publicly incorporated the GJMA as the command tower for private doctors as it needed cooperation from private doctors to implement the HI. The Japanese Medical Association (JMA) was thus implemented. Leaders in the GJMA had been hoping to expand their influence on fellow doctors. The HI, therefore, aligned the government's interest with the elite doctors' ambition.[14]

The power balance between the government and the JMA soon leaned in favor of the former. When the creation of the NHI was discussed in the mid-1930s, the JMA opposed it because it saw the NHI would be a new tool for the government to intervene in health care. When the war activities intensified, the JMA faced a robust enemy: the army. The army began to play a larger role in health care for the purpose of securing healthy soldiers for battlefields. Despite the JMA's opposition, the army successfully made the Fumimaro Konoe administration create a new health ministry and pass the NHI Act in the Imperial Diet. The JMA became politically defensive as its opposition was now labeled unpatriotic.

As both labor unions and doctors were absorbed into the government's war mobilization efforts, the government sought to expand the health insurance system. The Ministry of Health and Welfare (MHW) promoted the establishment of NHI associations. Soon after Japan started the war against the United

States and other Allied Powers in December 1941, the government took a radical step to rationalize the entire health care system, including the health care providers. In February 1942, the National Medical Care Act (Kokumin Iryō Hō) was enacted to create new public hospitals and clinics, regulate private hospitals, and reorganize the JMA as a state entity.

Meanwhile, the government expanded its power in health insurance to increase coverage and reduce the cost as much as possible. The HI was expanded to workers in smaller firms by reducing the requirement from ten to five employees. It also offered better benefits for the enrollees' dependents. To reduce cost, the government introduced the copayment and government-controlled fee-for-service payment systems. The NHI was also reformed to make the establishment of the NHI associations mandatory. Now doctors were required to be in a position where they would not be able to refuse to accept national health insurance.[15]

After serious air raids on the homeland began in mid-1944, the war became too devastating for the government to retain its investment in health care. Many medical facilities were damaged, and many of the NHI associations became dormant or even deceased. The quasi-universal health insurance system was built in haste for war purposes; therefore, it collapsed easily when the war failed. As to whether, how, and in what shape they might be revived after the war, it depended on the new postwar political situation. But the wartime experiences mattered as well.

The Cold War and Health Insurance Reforms

Japan accepted the Potsdam Declaration on August 15, 1945, and soon the US-led occupation began. It lasted until April 1952. In this nearly seven-year period, the General Headquarters of the Supreme Commander for the Allied Powers (hereafter GHQ) had the ultimate power to govern Japan, and health insurance reforms were shaped by the occupation authority. The GHQ saw the reform as part of its overall policy to demilitarize and democratize Japan. While the GHQ purged many politicians and bureaucrats who had been deeply engaged in the Japanese government's war activity, the Ministry of Health and Welfare was almost intact. The GHQ used the MHW bureaucrats to create and implement health care reforms by giving directions both formally and informally. In short, the GHQ officers from the United State shaped the course of reforms, and Japanese bureaucrats maintained the power against other domestic stakeholders by working together with the GHQ.[16]

The Cold War that started in the middle of the US-led occupation also contributed to the rise of conservative parties. In March 1947, the Truman Doctrine asserted that the United States would be the leader to defend the capitalism/liberal camp against the communist countries led by the Soviet Union. The GHQ gradually changed its stance toward Japan because the United States began to see Japan as an important front for anti-communism. Japan now needed to be economically developed to support the United States. Furthermore, the demilitarization policy began to be revised for the same purpose. The conservative parties and business groups gained political power in connection with this policy change by GHQ.

However, although the JMA and labor unions had been freed from the government's wartime restraints, they were still marginalized to influence health insurance policies. Theoretically, the GHQ's democratization policy could have empowered them to support the reforms, but in reality, they became obstacles to GHQ reforms for different reasons.

During the war, the JMA was turned into a state organization and doctors became part of the wartime regime. After the war, when the GHQ dissolved *zaibatsu*, the business conglomerates, it ended the state-run JMA as well. Instead, the JMA became a nongovernmental professional organization. However, the GHQ continued to view the even "democratized" JMA as a great hindrance to the GHQ's health care reform initiatives because the GHQ concluded that the Japanese healthcare system was outdated, and medical professionals were largely responsible for it.

The end of the war welcomed labor unions better than doctors. Labor unions were empowered by the GHQ's democratization policy. Many labor union leaders who were imprisoned during the war were freed. The labor movement gained momentum with the creation of new labor unions. On May 3, 1947, the new Constitution came into effect to support unions. Article 21 stipulated, "Freedom of assembly and association as well as speech, press and all other forms of expression are guaranteed."[17] However, the GHQ took a clear position to be anti-communist as the Cold War began to emerge. As the labor movement intensified with a general strike in January 1947, General MacArthur decided to ban the strike for fear of social unrest and Japan falling into the communist camp.

In order to understand the development of health insurance policy during the postwar reconstruction period, another factor to be considered is the institutional arrangements that had developed by the end of the war. They affected the stakeholders of the health insurance policy. There were two categories of public health insurance: employment-based health insurance and resident-based health insurance. The former's major program is the HI, and the latter is the NHI. They were different in structure, finance, and political power. Although the differences did not matter when the government had the dominant power, the postwar reform created opportunities for stakeholders to participate in the policymaking process and see their political advantages and disadvantages.

The SMHI of the HI required big companies to set up their own mutual societies to run programs based on their finances. The National Federation of Health Insurance Societies was the organization to represent all company-based health insurance societies. The GMHI, the other HI program, was a financially weaker program than the SMHI because employees of smaller companies tended to face more health risks owing to old age and engaging in more manual work. However, the HI's political strength was that the government was responsible for supervising as the regulator and administering the program as the insurer.

The NHI was inferior to the GMHI and the SMHI in terms of finance and political influence. The NHI's insurers were the NHI associations supervised by municipalities. Many of them were dormant during the postwar transition. The government subsided the administrative cost, but that was not enough for them to revive. The question was how to improve the health insurance system after the war. With the GHQ's strong power, the reform movement could have been directed to overhaul the entire system and build a new one. However, the GHQ's reform ended up improving the existing programs but maintaining the basic structure of the old health system. Although the GHQ was the primary actor to frame the discussion, the Japanese health officials ascertained the GHQ's basic stance to maintain their political leverage in the health insurance system.

The staff of the Section of Public Health and Welfare (PHW) in the GHQ were mostly former New Dealers who had a strong will to make changes in health insurance in the United States then and in Japan now.[18] Some of them were surprised to see Japan having what the United States did not have at that time: public health insurance programs that would potentially cover most of the population. But the programs needed improvement, even though some were better than others. Officers in the PHW considered integrating and rationalizing the programs. They were inspired by the Beveridge Plan proposed in 1944 to introduce an integrated national health insurance program for the entire population.[19]

The Beveridge Plan motivated Japanese scholars and bureaucrats as well. In March 1946, the Social Insurance Investigating Committee (Shakaihoshō Seido Chōsakai) was established by the MHW to review the social security system including health insurance. Particularly, reform-minded scholars pushed for the integration of the multiple programs. The new Japanese Constitution also encouraged them to propose a comprehensive social security system that resembled the Beveridge Plan.

While the integration issue was being discussed, GHQ conducted reforms to fix the existing programs to meet the Japanese people's demands. The NHI, which was the financially weakest program, was in crisis. The fee increase did not make up for the rapid inflation. As the NHI associations repeated back pays, doctors were not willing to accept NHI patients. The MHW tried to address the situation, but there was no easy way out. The fundamental problem was that many NHI associations were created by the government's wartime mobilization policy; their directors thought that the NHI expansion was a temporary measure, and they did not invest much to maintain it after the war.[20]

Some even proposed the abolishment of NHI. But the Section of the National Health Insurance (Kokumin Hoken Ka) of the MHW made a campaign to improve the NHI's finance and administration. In 1946, the government provided an additional 150-million-yen subsidy to the NHI. In June 1948, the NHI was reformed to shift its administrative responsibility from the NHI associations to municipalities. Therefore, each municipality would decide whether NHI associations were established or not.[21] Although it was not mandatory to set up associations, once decided, all residents must enroll. Mayors of cities and towns began to see the NHI as a venue to appeal to their constituencies.[22]

Just as the new NHI structure affected mayors' political behavior, the stakeholders in the HI began to voice their interest in the process of democratization as well. In particular, the National Federation of Health Insurance Societies began to push for the government to retain the existing structure by keeping the SMHI, financially the most robust program, as a separate program. Large companies worried that they would have more financial burden if the SMHI was merged into financially weaker programs. The Social Insurance Bureau (Hoken Kyoku) had promoted the integration idea since wartime, but the pressure of large companies made it adopt a more cautious attitude.[23]

The existing health insurance system also impacted labor unions. The labor movement first flourished through the support of GHQ's democratization policy. However, labor unions remained inactive in the health care issue. The labor movement was roughly divided into two groups. One was led by the Congress of Industrial Unions of Japan (Zennihon Sangyōbetu Rōdō Kumiai Kaigi, called Sanbetsu), which was supported by the Japanese Communist Party. It did not aim at negotiating to improve social programs with the government because this more radical movement at that time sought to overhaul capitalism and the existing political system.[24]

The other group is a moderate movement supported by the Socialist Party of Japan (SPJ), which was led by the Japanese Confederation of Labor Unions (Nihon Dōdō Kumiai Sōdōmei). This group included labor unions that were forcibly set up by the government in each company to mobilize for the war. As a result, they tended to focus on wage increases by individually negotiating with the employers. They cooperated with employers to enhance productivity and fought hard to increase income in the rapid inflation.[25] However, they did not focus on health insurance for three reasons.

The first was that they already had public health insurance coverage. Powerful labor unions were the ones in big companies. Workers in these unions had coverage by the financially strong SMHI. Employees in smaller companies were covered by the GMHI. The second reason was that health insurance was not yet used as a matter of fact. Although health insurance coverage expanded during the war, public health insurance did not become an essential part of people's lives and doctors' practices. In the period of super inflation and low national health insurance fee, many doctors returned to the tradition of private practice with a fee for service. There were many workers who either did not use their health insurance to see the doctors they needed or were unaware that they were covered under public health insurance. Third, many labor unions were not directly related to the most serious problem of the health insurance system: the NHI was financially and organizationally the weakest program. Because the NHI targeted the self-employed, labor unions were not interested in improving it. Therefore, the labor movement, including both the radical and the moderate wings, did not have a strong incentive to engage in the discussion of reforming the health insurance policy.

Like labor unions, doctors' associations were not active in the policymaking process of the health insurance policy, either. Soon after the occupation, GHQ directed the democratization of regional and national medical associations. The state-run JMA was dissolved and the JMA gained back its autonomy as a professional organization, but GHQ made sure that those who actively supported the government during the war would be expelled from leadership positions. Even with the new leaders, Crawford Sams, the head of the Section of Public Health and Welfare, was still skeptical about the JMA. He criticized the JMA for its excessive obsession with fee increases. He believed that the JMA should prioritize improving medical science and ethics.[26]

Sams was also disgusted about the fact that medical treatment and sales of medicine in Japan were not separated as much as he considered ideal. It was a long tradition that doctors in Japan diagnosed patients and prescribed and sold medicines. During the Tokugawa era, doctors were called *kusushi*, which literally meant pharmacists. They charged not for diagnosis but for medicine. The tradition continued in Japan while many contemporary Western countries saw doctors and pharmacists as different professionals. Although the Meiji government tried to follow the Western example, doctors in Japan were against the separation, which would significantly impact doctors' income negatively. Largely due to this history of the doctors' opposition, Sams saw the JMA as an obstacle to separating medical treatment and medical drug sales.[27] As a result, even after the JMA returned to the pre-war professional organization as GHQ directed, the JMA was still not welcomed by GHQ in the policymaking process.[28]

As political battles about the integration of the health insurance system continued, the Cold War began to impact GHQ's policy direction. In December 1948, the GHQ sent a direction to the Japanese government to stabilize the economy and become economically independent. A few months later, Joseph Dodge, former chairman of the Detroit Bank and now the financial advisor to General MacArthur, came to Japan to promote the stabilization plan. Deflation policy was one of those emphasized policies. The GHQ now focused on Japan's fiscal soundness and economic development by creating a strong capitalist alliance with the United States. As the policy shifted, it then became difficult for the government to increase the investment in health care policy.[29] The deflation policy helped conservative parties justify their cautious stance toward the welfare policy, but the Communist Party and the radical wing of the labor movement struggled to gain the public support of gaining seats in the Diet.

There appeared to still be hope left for nonconservative parties. In 1947, the SPJ succeeded in forming the cabinet with Tetsu Katayama as the prime minister, but it was not a single-party cabinet but was joined by the Democratic Party of Japan and the Japan Cooperative Party. Soon the SPJ lost its momentum. When the peace treaty was discussed and it became clear that Shigeru Yoshida, the prime minister from the Japan Liberal Party, planned to have the treaty without the Soviet Union, the SPJ was divided into two groups, mainly based on whether members would support the treaty plan or not. The Cold War made Japanese politics shift to the right. As a result, conservative parties backed by businesses were reluctant to make fundamental changes to the health insurance system.

When the US-led occupation ended in April 1952, the GHQ had made many significant changes in social policy areas. The Unemployment Insurance Act of 1947 and the Daily Life Assistance Act of 1950 were introduced. However, there were minimal changes in the field of health insurance. After the GHQ left Japan, the movement to achieve universal health care intensified, but the fragmented nature of the health insurance system largely influenced the political battles to maintain the status quo.

Universal Yet a Divided System

While the GHQ toned down its demand for radical reform, some Japanese scholars continued to push for it. The Advisory Council on Social Security (Shakaihoshō Seido Shingikai) was the space for them to do this. The council was in fact created by the GHQ's direction when there was still momentum for radical reform in the GHQ. In August 1947, the GHQ invited a group of social security specialists from the United States to make a detailed proposal for comprehensive reforms. The proposal included the establishment of an advisory council.

In December 1948, the Advisory Council was created as a powerful organization, which was composed of Diet members, government officials, insurer representatives, medical professionals, and scholars. Any decisions of the council had to be unanimous. The cabinet was required to consult the council on any significant changes in social security. Moreover, the Advisory Council was allowed to make any proposals to the cabinet without being asked. The first council president, Hyōe Ōuchi, who was an economist at the University of Tokyo, later became the advisor for the SPJ. The Advisory Council had a mission to create a comprehensive social security system for the future of a democratized Japan. Ōuchi said, "To make Japan a viable country, it is necessary to guarantee true social security for its individuals."[30] In October 1950, the Advisory Council made a "recommendation with respect to a social security system" (Shakaihoshōseido ni Kansuru Kankoku) to Prime Minister Shigeru Yoshida. It suggested that the NHI be financially improved by government subsidy and universal health care be established to make the uninsured participate in the NHI. However, the recommendation did not include the integration of health insurance programs.

What the Advisory Council recommended was different from the Beveridge Report, which was written by a single person. With varied interests on the council, it was relatively easy to agree on the broad and long-term goals of the Japanese social security system, but it was almost impossible to make a concrete unanimous proposal, as some stakeholders had contradicting interests.

Even the compromised proposal of the Advisory Committee faced chilly reception from the GHQ and the Japanese government because of their anti-communist stance during the process of writing the proposal. Seeing the proposal as the government's takeover of health care, the GHQ warned the government that the proposal would be considered "socialistic and it would not be appropriate financially."[31] The Yoshida administration, which was more in favor of economic development, did not take the proposals seriously.[32]

Meanwhile, the financial situation of the NHI became worse. Farmers' income improved in the postwar confusion, more specifically by the black market. But soon, this economic boom for farmers was over, and the deflation policy in the late 1940s deteriorated their financial situation. It was difficult for farmers to pay the NHI copayment, which was around 50 percent. Many also found it difficult to pay the premium. The municipalities that now had authority over the NHI pressured the government to expand its subsidy, but it was not easy.[33]

Both the NHI and the GMHI faced a financial crisis that began in 1948. The first reason for this was that more enrollees began to use their health insurance because GHQ's deflation policy made more people see health insurance as a safety net. Another reason was that many small companies began to make enrollees join the GMHI. As the number of self-pay patients decreased, more doctors started to accept health insurance enrollees. Consequently, the two programs faced financial difficulties.[34]

As the GMHI's finance deteriorated, labor unions began to push harder for the improvement of the social security system. The Congress of Industrial Unions of Japan (Zennihon Sangyōbetsu Rōdōkumiai Kaigi, CIU) took the lead. Backed by the Japan Communist Party, this left-wing labor union included organized medical staff who suffered from the low fee schedule.[35] The General Council of Trade Unions of Japan (Sōhyō), a more moderate labor union, also decided to participate in the movement. However, as Sōhyō was basically anti-communist, it had a delicate relationship with the CIU.[36]

The JMA sought to make a comeback as well to influence the policymaking process by utilizing this opportunity. The JMA leaders had seen its members complaining that the national health insurance fee did not increase to match the ongoing inflation. The JMA's main goal was to increase the national health insurance fee for its members' finance.

The JMA and labor unions were on the same page regarding pressurizing the government to stabilize the GMHI. The increase of national subsidy would benefit both, but they had varying interests regarding raising the fee schedule. It would be beneficial for the JMA as long as the premium and copayment did not become too high for workers to see doctors. However, increasing the fee had a nuanced meaning to the labor unions. As doctors, organized medical staff would be better off, but other union members tried to avoid paying higher premiums and copayments. This point of interest connected the labor unions with the government and business organizations that liked to lower health care costs. Therefore, whether the JMA and labor unions could get along depended on how to frame the national health insurance problem and how much the enrollees had to bear the financial burden. Soon the cooperation between the JMA and labor unions fell apart. It was Tarō Takemi who was largely responsible for this failure of cooperation.

Takemi served as the JMA's vice president twice in 1950 and 1952 and subsequently was elected as the president in 1957. He served in that position for 26 years until 1982. William Steslicke writes about Takemi's impact on the JMA:

> It was not until after the election of Taro Takemi as president in April 1957 ... that the JMA began to attract widespread attention and condemnation as an atsuryoku dantai (pressure group). It is only since Takemi's election and forceful leadership, moreover, that the JMA [became] of key importance in medical care administration and politics.[37]

Takemi rescued the JMA from a politically weak position by confronting the MHW bureaucrats and gaining material benefits for JMA members through direct negotiation with influential politicians of the Liberal Democratic Party (LDP).

Takemi's personal background mattered in his strategy. He was not a typical elite doctor. He dropped out of Keio University and eventually opened his own clinic in Ginza, a place close to the political center. Meanwhile, he gained strong connections in politics by marrying the granddaughter of Nobuaki Makino, an influential politician. Through this marriage, he also became a kin of Shigeru Yoshida, who served as the prime minister for about seven years from May 1946 to May 1947 and from October 1948 to December 1954.[38]

His personal connections in politics ensured that Takemi was picked first as the JMA's vice president. He met the expectation to help the JMA to get preferential tax treatment for doctors by negotiating directly with Finance Minister Hayato Ikeda, a disciple of Yoshida's. He understood that the best way to appeal to the JMA members was to bring direct material benefits, mostly higher national health insurance fees, to them. Rather than approaching the MHW's top bureaucrats who wielded significant power to set the fee schedule, he pressured the LDP politicians to change the way of business in the MHW to achieve his goal.

Pressing the government for material benefits was, of course, not particular to doctors. Other organizations in the private sector did that too. But what was unique about doctors was that the government defined significantly what medical services they should provide and how much they could charge for each service. Moreover, as described, the national health insurance fee did not catch up with the postwar inflation rate for many years. The JMA members understood that the JMA had been driven to a corner by the MHW bureaucrats along with the GHQ in the policymaking process. This was why JMA members elected Takemi with the hope of getting the better out of the bureaucrats.

To solidify his political base in the JMA, he strengthened his tie with the LDP. The 1950s was a good period not only for Takemi but also for the LDP. Right after the war, many political parties emerged with inclinations toward the right or the left. Katayama of the SPJ formed the cabinet once, but conservative parties controlled the cabinet the rest of the time. Two large conservative parties despite their names, the Liberal Party of Japan and the Democratic Party of Japan, merged after the 1955 House of Representative election into the LDP. After that, the SPJ remained the second-largest party in the Diet in the 1950s and 1960s, but their seats in the Diet trailed far behind the LDP's.[39]

Economic booms in the 1950s worked well for the LDP to remain powerful. The economic downturn due to the GHQ's deflation policy ended with the outbreak of the Korean War, a military confrontation of the enmity between the Soviet Union and the United States. Japan became an important supply base for the American military during the Korean War, which helped the recovery of its economy. From 1954 to 1957, Japan had a strong economic boom called Jinmu Boom (Jinmu Keiki). Jinmu is considered the first emperor of Japan. The term meant that the economic boom had been the strongest since the birth of the country. The government's economic white paper declared in 1956 that the "Postwar reconstruction is now over."[40]

In addition to the expansion of the economy, the LDP took another advantage of the Cold War international context. In 1951, the Treaty of San Francisco was signed by 49 countries to officially end the war between Japan and the Allied Powers. The Soviet Union did not sign it. The treaty demonstrated that Japan was clearly in the American camp. Prime Minister Yoshida went on to sign another treaty, the US–Japan Security Treaty, which allowed the American military base to remain in Japan. Left socialists opposed the treaties, but their movement could not significantly increase the support base. Instead, the LDP succeeded in enjoying the American stand by continuing to maintain its strong power economically and politically.

The preceding was the context in which the movement to introduce the universal health insurance system unfolded in the 1950s. By the time the occupation ended in April 1952, the introduction of universal health care appeared inevitable. The prevalent question was when and how it was going to be done.

The GMHI faced financial crisis again soon after the short recovery during the Korean War. In 1954, the GMHI had a large deficit, resulting in late payments to doctors.[41] The government tried to deal with the problem but was criticized for playing favorites with workers enrolled in the GMHI while ignoring people who did not have health insurance coverage at all.[42]

In April 1955, the government set up a seven-member committee to research the financial needs of the national health insurance programs. In July 1956, the MHW established another committee to clarify that universal health care was necessary for Japan. Its report included a proposal that all municipalities were required to administer the NHI.[43]

The push for universal health care, however, did not have a strong movement to integrate the multiple programs. The British-style single-payer program was beyond discussion. The question was how to cover the uninsured with the existing framework. The fragmented structure of national health insurance had made stakeholders try to protect and maximize their own material benefits in the given institutional setting.

There were two groups among the uninsured. One was the self-employed, such as farmers in municipalities that had not set up an NHI association. It would be a logical solution to make it mandatory for all municipalities to form NHI associations. The other group was employees in small companies with fewer than five workers. In this case, it was more difficult to decide on an ideal solution. Some claimed that, as it did in the past, the GMHI should increase its coverage to include these people. Others argued that a similar program should be established specifically for this group. Health insurance for micro-enterprise workers, they argued, was difficult to administer.

The conclusion was that the existing employment-based programs remained as they were, and the NHI was to be expanded to cover the rest of the population. In 1958, the NHI Act was amended to make it mandatory for municipalities to administer the NHI, increase the national subsidy, and standardize the copayment.[44]

The national subsidy had been 20 percent of the program cost. The amendment introduced an adjusting subsidy by which the financially better national health insurance associations could have additional subsidies up to 5 percent. The copayment had varied depending on municipalities, but now the amendment standardized it to 50 percent. Those improvements, however, did not narrow the gap between the NHI and the employment-based programs much, although major stakeholders accepted the change more or less positively.

JMA president Takemi had focused on gaining immediate material benefits for the members and holding authority against the MHW bureaucrats by negotiating with influential LDP politicians. Because he sensed that it would be hard to reverse the movement toward the introduction of universal health care, he tried to make the best out of it. He achieved sufficient fee increases and gained compromises from the government to loosen regulations on doctors.

Big businesses were happy with the fact that universal health care was introduced without changing the SMHI programs they ran. The extension of the NHI to the rest of the population did not hurt the SMHI's finance. Employers could continue to enjoy having the SMHI to appease labor unions, as it was obvious that the SMHI was a much better program.

Labor unions did not have a strong influence compared with the JMA and big businesses. Many of them allied with the SPJ, the second-largest party. The SPJ, however, had only limited influence on the overall reform debate. When policy options were brought to the table in the assigned committee in the Diet, all the major stakeholders had already agreed upon the arrangement and there was not much that the SPJ could change.[45] Moreover, the interests of

SPJ and unions and did not conflict with that of the JMA and big businesses because labor unions in big companies had an interest in protecting the SMHI.[46]

Conclusion

The late 1940s and early 1950s were the periods when Japan moved toward universal health care. The movement overlapped with the early period of the Cold War. When China was taken by the Chinese Communist Party, and the Korean Peninsula became an actual battlefield of the two camps of the Cold War, the United States took the lead in promoting the capitalist world. In Japan, the United States was the final decision maker during the military occupation from 1945 to 1952. The Cold War significantly impacted the shift of direction in health insurance reforms in Japan.

The reform during the Cold War did not change the basic structure of Japan's old health insurance system. Rather, it played a role in solidifying it. The structural foundation came from the legacy of wartime government that made health policy through the top-down approach. To the GHQ, the JMA, which was absorbed into the government's war mobilization, was responsible for the backwardness of Japan's health care, not the MHW bureaucrats who more directly contributed to the wartime policies. After the occupation ended, the JMA under Takemi's leadership began to influence the policymaking process by negotiating directly with influential politicians. In doing so, the JMA gained immediate material benefits, such as fee increases, but not fundamental reforms of the system. Takemi, however, had to compromise with the LDP politicians whom the big businesses had a major influence on. Big businesses and moderate labor unions in big companies shared an interest in keeping the HI, especially the SMHI for their benefits. More radical labor unions backed by the Communist Party of Japan were marginalized. In the end, Japan achieved universal health care with the wartime policy legacy remaining almost intact.

Notes

1 For an analysis of the longer-term development of health insurance policy and politics with historical institutionalism, see Takakazu Yamagishi, *Health Insurance Politics in Japan: Policy Development, Government, and the Japan Medical Association* (Ithaca, NY: Cornell University Press, 2022).

2 Before 1961, there were other employment categories that the HI did not deal with. For example, public employees and private school teachers were allowed to establish their own mutual associations. These programs also had institutional and political implications, but owing to limited space, this chapter does not focus on them.

3 Yoshihara Kenji and Wada Masaru, *Nihon Iryōhoken Seidoshi* [History of Japanese health insurance] (Tokyo: Tōyō Keizai Shuppansha, 1999), 125.

4 According to Japanese custom, I have adopted the order of surname first and given name last for Japanese publications. Otherwise, the order is first name and last name.

118 *Takakazu Yamagishi*

5 For the establishment of the HI, see Kitahara Ryūji, *Kenkōhoken to Ishikai: Shakai-hoken Sōshiki niokeru Ishi to Iryō* [The health insurance system and the JMA: Doctors and medicine at the beginning of social health insurance] (Tokyo: Tōshindō, 1999).

6 Kōseishō Imu Kyoku, *Isei Hyakunen* [One-hundred-year history of medicine] (Tokyo: Gyōsei, 1976), 222.

7 The implementation was delayed due to the Great Kantō earthquake in 1923.

8 For the study that examines the relationship between the war mobilization and health insurance policy, see Shō Kashin, *Nihongata Fukushi Kokka no Keisei to Jūgonen Sensō* [The fifteen–year war and the formation of the Japanese welfare state] (Kyoto: Minerva Shobō, 1998); Gregory J. Kasza, *One World of Welfare: Japan in Comparative Perspective* (Ithaca, NY: Cornell University Press, 2006); Takakazu Yamagishi, *War and Health Insurance Policy in Japan and the United States* (Baltimore: Johns Hopkins University Press, 2011).

9 Ōkouchi Kazuo, "Nihon Rōdo7shi ni okeru Mondai to Hōhō [Problems and Solutions in the Japanese Labor Movement History]," Ōkouchi Kazuo and Fujita Wakao eds. *Nihon no Rōdōmondai IV Rōdōkumiai Undōshi* [History of Labor Union Movement] (Tokyo: Kōbundō, 1972), 3–5.

10 They included the one led by Bunji Suzuki, who worked closely with Sakuzō Yoshino.

11 Margaret Powell and Masahira Anesaki, *Health Care in Japan* (London: Routledge, 1990), 30.

12 Kawakami Takeshi, *Gendai Nihon Iryōshi* [History of modern Japanese health care] (Tokyo: Keisō Shobō, 1965), 155; Ogawa Kenzō, *Igaku no Rekishi* (Tokyo: Chūōkōron Shinsha, 1964), 211–12.

13 Sugaya Akira, *Nihon Iryō Seidoshi* [History of Japanese medical institutions] (Tokyo: Hara Shobō, 1976), 109–7.

14 Ikura Yasumasa, *Shindan Takemi Tarō* [Evaluating Takemi Tarō] (Tokyo: Sōshisha, 1979), 50.

15 Kōseishō Gojūnenshi Henshū Iinkai, *Kōseishō Gojūnenshi: Kijutsu Hen* [Fifty-year history of the Ministry of Welfare, description volume] (Tokyo: Chūō Hōki Shuppan, 1988), 545–48.

16 For how the occupation took place and impacted Japan, see John Dower, *Embracing Defeat: Japan in the Wake of World War II* (New York: W. W. Norton, 1999).

17 Prime Minister of Japan and His Cabinet, "The Constitution of Japan," https://japan.kantei.go.jp/constitution_and_government_of_japan/constitution_e.html, accessed on June 6, 2022.

18 For how American politics affected health insurance reforms in Japan, see Adam D. Sheingate and Takakazu Yamagishi, "Occupation Politics: American Interests and the Struggle over Health Insurance in Postwar Japan," *Social Science History* 30, no. 1 (Spring 2006).

19 The Beveridge Plan was written by William Beveridge, a highly regarded economist and Liberal politician. He released a report calling for a progressive and comprehensive social security reform. It advocated free universal health care funded by central government taxation.

20 Nakashizuka Michi, *Iryōhoken no Gyōsei to Seiji, 1895–1954* [Administration and Politics of Health Insurance, 1895–1954] (Tokyo: Yoshikawa Kōbundō, 1998), 297.

21 Nakashizuka, *Iryōhoken no Gyōsei to Seiji, 1895–1954*, 298.

22 Arioka Jirō, *Sengo Iryō no Gojūnen: Iryōhoken Seido no Butaiura* [Fifty years of postwar medical care: Behind the scenes in the health insurance system] (Tokyo: Nihon Iji Shinpōsha, 1997), 109.

23 Nakashizuka, *Iryōhoken no Gyōsei to Seiji, 1895–1954*, 296.

24 Kume Ikuo, *Rōdō Seiji: Sengoseiji nonakano Rōdōkumiai* [Labor Politics: Labor Unions in the Post-WWII] (Chūkōshinsho, 2005), 149–50.
25 Kume, *Rōdō Seiji*, 154.
26 Nakashizuka, *Iryōhoken no Gyōsei to Seiji, 1895–1954*, 302.
27 In 1956, the Separation of Medical Treatment and the Sale of Medicines Act began to be implemented, but the JMA succeeded in making many exceptions, and doctors, in fact, continued drug dispensation.
28 For Sams's view on Japanese health care, see Crawford Sams, *Medic: The Mission of an American Military Doctor in Occupied Japan and Wartorn Korea* (New York: Routledge, 1998).
29 Yoneyuki Sugita, *Japan's Shifting Status in the World and the Development of Japan's Medical Insurance System* (Singapore: Springer, 2019), 219, 224.
30 Yoshihara and Wada, *Nihon Iryōhoken Seidoshi*, 134.
31 Ibid., 137.
32 Sugita, *Japan's Shifting Status in the World and the Development of Japan's Medical Insurance System*, 207–8.
33 Nakashizuka, *Iryōhoken no Gyōsei to Seiji, 1895–1954*, 308–309.
34 Ibid., 306–308.
35 Ibid., 314.
36 Taishirō Shirai, "Nippon Rōdōkumiai Sōdōmei no Undō [Movement of Japanese Federation of Labour], 145–46, in Ōkouchi and Fujita eds. *Nihon no Rōdōmondai IV*. Sōhyō was established in 1950 in response to the creation of the Japan Federation of Employers' Association (Nihon Keieisha Dantai Renmei, Nikkeiren) in 1948. It sought to exclude the power of labor unions from company management. Kume, 157–59.
37 William E. Steslicke, *Doctors in Politics: The Political Life of the Japan Medical Association* (New York: Columbia University Press, 1973), 46.
38 For the detailed personal background of Takemi, see Takakazu Yamagishi, "A Short Biography of Takemi Taro, the President of the Japan Medical Association," *Journal of the Nanzan Academic Society Social Sciences* 1 (January 2011): 49–56.
39 In the 1958 election, the LDP had 287 and the SPJ had 166; in 1960, the LDP 296/the SPJ 145; in 1963, the LDP 283/the SPJ 144; in 1967, the LDP 277/the SPJ 140; in 1969, the LDP 288/the SPJ 90. For the party politics after the war, https://dl.ndl.go.jp/view/download/digidepo_999897_po_065104.pdf?contentNo=1, accessed on June 9, 2022.
40 Yoshihara and Wada, *Nihon Iryōhoken Seidoshi*, 140.
41 Tsuchida Takeshi, "Kokumin Kaihoken 50nen no Kiseki [Trajectory of 50-year History of the Universal Health Care]," *Shakaihoshō Kenkyū* 47, no. 3 (Winter 2011): 245.
42 Arioka, *Sengo Iryō no Gojūnen*, 105.
43 "Dainiji Sekai Taisengo no Iryō Hoken Seido wo meguru Ugoki, Part 2 [Post-WWII Environment regarding the Health Insurance System]," *Kōsei no Shihyō* 64, no. 4 (April 2017): 43, https://www.hws-kyokai.or.jp/images/book/chiikiiryo-9.pdf, accessed on June 3, 2022.
44 "Dainiji Sekai Taisengo no Iryō Hoken Seido wo meguru Ugoki," 44.
45 Yuki Yasuhiro, *Fukushishakai ni okeru Iryō to Seiji: Shinryōhoshu wo meguru Kankeidantai no Ugoki* [Medicine and politics in the welfare society: Activities of interest groups regarding the fee schedule] (Tokyo: Honnoizumisha, 2004), 41.
46 Ikegami Naoki and John Campbell, *Nihon no Iryō: Tosei to Baransu Kankaku* [Health care in Japan: Control and sense of balance] (Tokyo: Chuko Shinsho, 1996), 30.

5 Foreign Aid, Virus Research and Preventive Medicine in India during the Cold War, 1950–1962

Shirish N. Kavadi

Introduction

This chapter studies the foreign aid of virus research and preventive medicine in independent India during the early Cold War when both the US and the USSR competed to extend their influence through development aid and professional assistance to the newly independent countries. International organizations such as the World Health Organization (WHO) and the Rockefeller Foundation (RF) played important roles in shaping global health and medical research in India via technical and financial assistance. The chapter focuses on the RF's support for the virus research program in India with a brief introduction of the general background of the internationalization of public health and medical research and the transformation of global health that coincided with the decolonization and independence of India. Vijay Kumar Chattu and W. Andy Knight have highlighted "global health diplomacy" as a major facet of the internationalization of public health. It is also part of public diplomacy followed by nations. Global health diplomacy is sometimes interchangeably used with the terms *medical diplomacy, disease diplomacy* and *vaccine diplomacy*.[1] These terms pertain to both therapeutic and prophylactic medicine. Although these terms are not explicitly used in the chapter, they are implicit in the discussion of the development of virus research and preventive measures to eradicate and control virus-related communicable and infectious diseases in India.

Scholarly studies on preventive policy and public health programs in India have discussed four various approaches: (1) the community approach that is directed at addressing the social and economic basis of ill health of a community, (2) training medical doctors in preventive and social medicine and health personnel at a lower level in the implementation of public health principles and practices, (3) the technocratic approach that relies on technical methods to eradicate and control communicable and infectious diseases, and (4) the exploration of the nature and transmission of diseases via field investigation and laboratory.[2] All four dimensions can exist together but may not balance out, and there may be lop-sidedness in overall health policy. However, inadequate attention has been given to the development of medical research in preventive medicine that includes virus research and the creation of health knowledge and

DOI: 10.4324/9781003318163-6

disease control. The WHO and other transnational and international organizations have supported most of the virus research for preventive medicine. For the WHO, India epitomized the range of conditions in what would be, during the 1950s, characterized as the underdeveloped world.[3]

Public health and preventive medicine had been a deeply contested theme during the colonial period and remained so after India's independence. Nehru's conviction in science and technology defined his idea of "state science," which meant that scientific research was to be conducted at state direction and discretion.[4] According to David Arnold, Nehru did not favor "ivory tower" research, with scientists working in seclusion for personal intellectual fulfillment; instead, he believed that scientists "had to accept the logic of funding resources controlled by the state and state-driven science policy."[5] Nehru's vision was shared and supported by India's most gifted scientists. Protagonists of national science suggested an ecosystem that appeared favorable to medical science, and yet as Arnold points out, Nehru's passion for science and technology did not extend to medical science, which had a biased and unfavorable bearing on the development of health and medicine.[6] There was continuity in the parsimonious colonial policy of underinvestment in health and medicine. Foreign aid appeared as a necessity for health and medical programs that led the Indian government and agencies to seek aid from both the superpowers as they competed to extend their influence on the third world in which India had a pivotal place.

Virus research in India was an essential aspect of the advancement of medical science and the creation and sharing of medical knowledge crucial to preventive medicine and public health. This study investigates the RF's support for medical research and especially virus research in India by founding the Virus Research Centre (VRC) in Poona (now Pune), one of seven field laboratories the RF established worldwide. Today, it is known as the National Institute of Virology (NIV) and is India's premier virology research institute. The discussion details the RF's global virus program, its reasons for setting up the VRC in India in 1952, and the objectives and scope of the program. The examination of these topics will help us understand the serological investigations and the surveys the VRC undertook during the first decade of its establishment and the inquiries it conducted on behalf of the Indian government into the epidemics that broke out during those years.

The Indian response to American and RF's aid was mixed and, at times, contradictory.[7] The work of the VRC was questioned and suspicions articulated in certain Indian quarters, particularly among left-leaning Indians with anti-American sentiments and the communists. The various controversies indicated the bearing the Cold War had on the RF (American) presence and its activities in India. The chapter focuses on the period from 1948 to 1962 when international health and support from abroad to India's medical research were heavily influenced by the Cold War conflict. Also, in 1962, Dr. T. Ramchandra Rao was appointed the first Indian director of the center, although the official RF association would end only in the early 1970s.

Internationalization and Politicization of Medicine

Disease, public health and medicine have been internationalized, politicized and militarized since the mid-nineteenth century facilitated by pandemic threats and the global circulation of medical knowledge through transnational studies of diseases and collaboration among medical scientists. International organizations, both private and public, sponsored public health campaigns with the support of extensive personnel, material and financial resources. Public health and medicine no longer remained matters of domestic policies even as questions were raised about state responsibility for public health. Medical care and financial demands were made on national governments when epidemics and quarantines disrupted and threatened trade, commerce, industrial activity and social life. The imposition of quarantines was not always welcomed by either the government or the common people.

The discovery of bacteria and viruses and the emergence of laboratory medicine and germ theory in the nineteenth century brought a paradigm shift to medical science. Individuals, as well as teams of medical scientists, from different nationalities undertook investigations into the etiology, pathology and epidemiology of diseases most prominently cholera, plague, malaria, influenza, hookworm and yellow fever, among others, and conducted research into and testing of vaccines at various geographical locations. Those investigations were as much motivated by scientific curiosity and public health concerns as personal glory and nationalist pride. The appearance of tropical medicine as a specialization and the establishment of schools of tropical medicine in Europe, North and Latin America gave momentum to this international endeavor.

In the post–World War II (WWII) years, health became central to the idea of national development, with the Cold War international aid to promote development and public health suggested as a way to counter the spread of communism.[8] Marcos Cueto observes in the context of Latin America that through the 1940s and 1950s, the language, policies and activities of international health by new bilateral and multilateral organizations were profoundly shaped by the Cold War. He argues that international health was "validated as an important tool of foreign and economic policy by a web of multilateral, bilateral and philanthropic institutions."[9] International health became a tool for "the growing importance of American hegemony in medical and scientific proposals for developing countries and to the organization and use of a web of bilateral and multilateral agencies."[10]

The US and RF took the initiative in setting up international health organizations such as the WHO modeled on the RF itself and influenced its approach to global health.[11] The US, as Gary Hess notes, turned the WHO into a "captive of US political interests" and used its own approach of health matters to guide the WHO.[12] The result was that instead of addressing the basic economic and social causes of diseases and the weaknesses of health systems of developing countries, the WHO relied on technology and directed its own interventions as a simple tool of "technical assistance" in the world. Those techno-centric campaigns targeted infectious and communicable diseases such as malaria, smallpox, and others.[13] The WHO set up a virology program in Spain in 1951, while influenza networks were developed across countries after the Influenza Center was created in 1947 in London.[14] The WHO's Global Pandemic Influenza Action Plan was a further example of vaccine diplomacy. Cueto has underlined that the WHO's approach consisted of "a limited program of disease control" and was essentially technocratic in nature.[15] He notes WHO's "New technical disease-oriented intervention and administration schemes were funded by Western industrial societies" and then extended to developing countries.[16] Its outcome, according to Cueto was that "Technical assistance allowed the economic and social realities that led to underdevelopment to be ignored, because it was based on the idea that transferring knowledge of science and technology was the key to development."[17]

Referring to more recent times, Tim Adams observes: "The World Health Organization has argued for years that the mechanics of our globalised economy, the dramatic increase in urbanisation and mass intercontinental travel has exponentially increased the chances for infectious disease to mutate and spread."[18] The WHO identified a record 1,100 "worldwide epidemic events" between 2002 and 2007. He quotes Frank Snowden: "Their names now run the gamut from A to Z – from avian flu to Zika, and scientists caution that far more potentially dangerous pathogens exist than have so far been discovered."[19] Snowden argues that the old wisdom that saved human societies in the past must be brought to the front and center of government. Public health must be the highest law, and all else follows from it.[20]

The WHO drafted and adopted the International Health Regulations (IHR) in 2005 to monitor and address health threats arising from emerging infectious diseases. Medical diplomacy, which is a part of public diplomacy, involves teamwork and alliance among countries to work concurrently on attaining health goals. The one that concerns this chapter the most is the vaccine diplomacy that is engaged with the utilization and delivery of vaccines. Chattu and Knight observe:

> Unlike the other aspects of medical or public health interventions, vaccines are unique as they are the single most potent intervention ever developed by humankind in terms of the number of lives they save. Vaccine science diplomacy is a unique hybrid of global health and science diplomacy that could lead to the development and testing of some highly innovative neglected disease vaccines.[21]

In the early Cold War, the Soviet Union stayed out of the WHO from 1948 to 1956 due to ideological differences with the US over socialized medicine and other issues. For the USSR, the WHO was not a conduit for offering aid to developing countries. In 1958, the Soviet Union sent a representative to the World Health Assembly and joined the WHO thereafter to collaborate on various preventive health programs. Amid the Cold War, the US and the USSR

worked jointly to eradicate smallpox, with the US providing much of the funding while the USSR offering the vaccine it had developed and successfully used
against smallpox in its own country.[22] Referring to the joint venture between
the two in developing the polio vaccine, Chattu and Knight point out:

> Vaccine science diplomacy entered the golden age during the Cold War
> between the U.S. and USSR that resulted in the development of an oral
> polio vaccine and a joint scientific collaboration between Dr. Albert Sabin
> (U.S.) and Dr. Mikhail Chumakov (USSR).[23]

This is significant as seen in the subsequent section that despite political differences, the US and the USSR worked jointly on matters relating to global health
security from the late 1950s. Vaccine diplomacy has manifested in international
efforts to ensure universal and equitable access for developing countries to vaccines for diseases that are likely to lead to pandemics. The RF's global virus
research program in India needs to be reevaluated for its importance in this
context.

The Cold War, Foreign Aid and Preventive Medicine in Independent India

On the eve of India's independence, two Committee Reports discussed public
health and medical planning for post-independence India. The National Planning Committee of the Indian National Congress set up a Health Sub-Com-
mittee headed by Major General Sir S. S. Sokhey, a member of the Indian
Medical Service, director of the Bombay-based Haffkine Institute and a past RF
medical fellow with training in the US. His report of 1948 stressed a commu-
nity-based primary care approach. The other was the government-appointed
Health Survey and Development Committee as part of its "Post-War Reconstruction Programme" headed by Sir Joseph Bhore, a member of the elite
Indian Civil Service.[24] Its report of 1946 recommended public health training,
rural public health and preventive programs for communicable and infectious
disease control and eradication but placed emphasis on medical education and
research. The latter in particular was strongly emphasized and supported by
bilateral and multilateral aid agencies after independence.[25]

At the time of India's independence in 1947, the international order faced
new challenges. The world was largely divided into the American and the
Soviet blocs in an emerging Cold War. India, which had just become independent, was cautious and wary in its approach to this new conflict. India
came up with the idea of nonalignment, refusing to be allied with either of the
two camps. Nonetheless, as Manu Bhagavan observes that India was posi-
tioned between the US and USSR blocs that were "truly global in scope" and
India's role was not minimal.[26] Sunil Amrith points out that during this period
and particularly through the 1950s Asia was at the center of international
efforts to free the world of disease, and India was at the core of the pan-Asian

and global debates about these endeavors. Moreover, India was located between "the history of Asian nationalism and decolonization", and the "history of postcolonial public health and medicine" making international institutions the location for the exchange of ideas and policies on disease, welfare and development.[27] The exchanges led to forging of intellectual, technological and personal connections.

David Engerman similarly argues that the two superpowers used foreign aid for development, modernization and health as a tool of the Cold War during the 1950s and 1960s and that India, the first and the largest of the colonies to become independent from Britain, was at the center of American and Soviet aid competition. On the recipient side, Engerman notes how nuclear scientists such as Homi Bhabha, a close adviser to Nehru, believed that "[n]ations like India should invoke the Cold War 'battle for hearts and minds' to obtain more aid on better terms—meaning lower prices, cheaper financing, and fewer restrictions on use." Foreign assistance, in the end, "came about through the efforts of different groups of policy makers, not necessarily through the government of India, to utilize their connections to advance their own economic visions and interests."[28]

The US offered fairly generous aid and assistance to independent India, recognizing its importance in the fight against communism.[29] Outside the Americas, India was the largest recipient of the RF's assistance covering health, medicine and community development and support to developing the Humanities in its universities in the broader context of the Cold War.[30] India relied on its nonalignment policy to welcome and receive foreign aid, even as suspicion about American intentions and motives was common in both the government circles and the public. India's different responses revealed the dilemma and inconsistency. Attitudes toward the US and Americans were mixed and sometimes contradictory. There was a tremendous attraction of the US, particularly its universities and the advancement in science, technology and medicine, which drew many Indian students to that country.[31] There were anti-American sentiments as well because of the various military blocs it built around India and its support to Pakistan.

In contrast, the Soviet Union maintained a certain distance by offering negligible bilateral aid that included exporting wheat to India. Joseph Stalin was suspicious and distrustful of Jawaharlal Nehru, India's first prime minister, whom he did not consider a revolutionary. Nehru had a strained relationship with Indian communists through whom the USSR attempted to exercise influence over its foreign policy. The situation changed after Stalin died and Nikita Khrushchev, first secretary of the Soviet Communist Party and who, in 1958, became the premier of USSR, declared the policy of "peaceful co-existence" with the West.[32] The change of policy however, did not necessarily ease Nehru's relations with the Indian communists who themselves were divided about supporting Nehru. Some supported Nehru because he showed certain socialist leanings, but others opposed him because they saw him as another bourgeois leader.[33] There was mutual distrust between Nehru and India's Communist

Party. Soviet aid from the mid-1950s was primarily directed at large infrastructure projects such as dams and hydroelectric plants that Nehru referred to as "temples of modern India" and public sector enterprises such as the pharmaceutical and drug industry.[34] The Soviet Union contributed to the building of the Indian Institute of Technology (IIT) in Bombay (now Mumbai), but it was unable to provide English-speaking teachers to Indian universities and research centers.[35] Ironically, many of the early teachers at the Bombay IIT were Americans.

The RF and the Virus Research in India: A New International Program

The RF underwent significant internal reorganization soon after World War II with important decisions about the scope and priorities of its future programs for the new international order that was shaped by the emerging Cold War, the decolonization and independence of countries in Asia and Africa and, most important, the policies of the two rival blocs toward the newly independent and developing countries. As part of the reorganization, the Trustees and senior officials decided to reorient the RF's worldwide health and medical program. The International Health Division (IHD) was dissolved in 1951 and other divisions such as the Division of Medicine and Public Health (DMPH) created to concentrate on medical education and research in developing countries.[36] The RF's policies and programs were not directly tied up with the US government's foreign policy but reflected the values and concerns of the policy in its dealings with developing countries in order to counter communism.

The RF, through its IHD, had a long history of health intervention in India. It made initial entry into British India and some of the independent Indian princely states in 1919. The RF believed that a main cause of worldwide poverty was infectious diseases that undermined productivity and hence became the target of its public health program. The RF carried on a global hookworm campaign from the Americas to Australia, and India was identified as the source of hookworm in the British colonies in South and Southeast Asia as well as Mauritius and the West Indies. Indentured Indian laborers on plantations in the colonies and free Indian migrants were identified as carriers of the disease. The RF set up public health departments and rural demonstration health units. It conducted public health awareness campaigns and malaria control and created the All India Institute of Hygiene and Public Health (AIIHPH) in India.[37] In the 1940s, apart from four field offices in Latin America, India was the only country to have an RF field office. The RF shifted to provide technical and financial support for virus research in post-independent India. The RF acknowledged that in tropical and semitropical regions insect-borne viruses were persistently active and thrived throughout the year owing to the unvarying and perpetual presence of mosquitoes and vulnerable animals like monkeys and mammals such as bats.[38]

The RF's virus research was an integral part of its IHD's insect-borne virus diseases program.[39] The IHD started virus studies on yellow fever in 1916 that were subsequently spurred on by the 1918 influenza pandemic. The tropics were believed to function like reservoirs, from which viruses were seasonally spread by migratory birds, bats and animals to cause eruptions of severe diseases in other temperate zones. Medical scientists were interested in investigating whether viruses infested cooler regions each summer from the tropics or whether viruses present in resident species were reactivated by the change of weather.[40]

The IHD had gathered a group of highly efficient and skilled personnel of medical research with equipment for tracking down special diseases and identifying arboviruses. In 1949, the IHD decided to expand its virus research by collecting new and potentially dangerous arboviruses. The program, which aimed at isolating and classifying these viruses in order to further understand their biology, comprised scientists trained in clinical virology, pathology, immunology and epidemiology. From 1949 and 1952, intensive studies showed evidence of a close relationship between some of the newly discovered viruses and the well-known causative agents of human disease.[41] The studies convinced IHD officials that a systematic investigation of the distribution and epidemiology of the arthropod-borne virus diseases, pathogenic for humans and domestic animals, should become a part of its program. Before it was dissolved, the IHD set up a special committee to explore the possibilities for the RF to undertake a continuous and long-term engagement of an international virus research program on arthropod-borne virus diseases.

In the 1950s and early 1960s, the RF set up seven field laboratories or stations in six countries on four continents. An important aspect of the field laboratories was that each of them was encouraged to keep the other groups informed of the work they were doing in order to stimulate discussion and comment. In the field laboratories, attention was focused primarily on the epidemiological aspects of the arboviruses that involved humans, animals, and birds, as well as the vector mosquitoes, ticks and sandflies. The work of these field stations was coordinated with the New York–based RF Virus Laboratory (RFVL). Additionally, informal collaboration was developed with laboratories maintained by other organizations, namely, close liaison was established with the US Army–run General Medical Laboratory in Tokyo, the Medical Research Laboratory in Kuala Lumpur and units of the US Public Health Service.[42]

Creation of a Virus Research Center for India

The RF chose India as part of its global virus program and linked the research there with a network of activities at other research sites. This renewed interest on the part of the RF in virology seemed opportune for both the RF and India. Dr. C. G. Pandit, secretary of the Indian Council of Medical Research (ICMR), was director of the King Institute at Guindy, Madras, in the 1930s and 1940s.[43] He had run a small unit for the study of filterable viruses at Guindy. He had also been a recipient of a Rockefeller Fellowship and spent time in the New York Laboratory, studying yellow fever and the development of a yellow fever vaccine. With his departure from the King Institute, the virus research there came to a halt. Pandit had plans to revive investigations into virology under the aegis of the ICMR. In 1950, when George Strode, director of the IHD, was on a visit to India, Pandit informally discussed with him the status of virus research in India and inquired about the possibility of aid and assistance from the RF to develop a virus research program if the ICMR could come up a definite plan.[44]

The then Health Minister Rajkumari Amrit Kaur, who respected Pandit for his research work, suggested that he use the surplus funds left with the ICMR from before independence to set up laboratory facilities to conduct his own research. Pandit declined the offer and instead suggested that the funds be used to build up the ICMR as an active research organization for promoting medical research in India. He thought the funds could become useful in giving the scheme of a virus research center a substantive form.[45] The ICMR under Pandit had already made a start by establishing a research unit on polio in Bombay.

The RF agreed that India presented the best opportunity for establishing a field laboratory.[46] Max Theiler, who headed the Rockefeller Foundation Virus Laboratory (RFVL) in New York, identified India as offering the greatest potential for virus research. Telford Work, an RF official and the second director of the VRC, echoed the colonial portrayal of India as the biggest laboratory for research in tropical diseases by describing it as "a fertile field of unexplored virus problems" and "a paradise for biologists."[47] RF officials were of the opinion that the Indian program would "have a definite objective of developing permanent diagnostic and research facilities."[48]

H. Smith, associate director of the RF, and Theiler toured India in March and April 1951, visiting Bombay, Poona, Bangalore, Coonoor, Madras, Calcutta and Delhi for the purpose of setting up a virus research program.[49] They met senior Indian officials, particularly those who had relations with the RF, such as RF past fellows. They had a stopover in Geneva to meet Sokhey, then a vice director at the WHO. In India, they met KC.K.E Raja, also a former RF fellow, who was the health secretary of India at the time.[50] They met Pandit, an "old and good friend of ours" and who "had done the only significant virus work in the country and was more intimately familiar with opportunities for virus research than anyone else."[51] In addition they had meetings with Kaur and Colonel C. K. Lakshmanan, the director-general of health services. These were people whose opinions would matter the most in the virus research program.

Smith and Theiler were impressed with what they saw and felt that there was a great need for such studies "not only to clarify health problems in India, but to complete the world epidemiological picture of many virus disease."[52] It was proposed that the program "would be a cooperative undertaking to foster epidemiological studies on virus diseases in India where virus infection had not yet received sufficient attention and hence appeared a field worth cultivating."[53] The program would be primarily concerned with investigating arboviruses or viruses transmitted by bloodsucking arthropods and the study of virus diseases in humans that were transmitted by these arthropods. There were certain kinds of virus research that would be outside the scope of the VRC as Robert Watson, RF representative in India, pointed out to Pandit, "I think it should be emphasized that the work will not be related to measles, influenza, smallpox, rabies and, particularly, anterior poliomyelitis; only to unexplored fields of virus research, which never before has been attempted in India."[54] Poona was selected as the location for the VRC because of the suitable climate that was very important to ensure proper breeding and maintenance of a mouse colony and the convenience of logistics with the city readily accessible by air and rail to facilitate investigations of viral epidemics occurring in different regions of India. It provided suitable laboratory space with the availability of housing for staff and auxiliary medical institutions.[55] The Government of Bombay offered accommodations for the center in a vacant two-storied building that had formerly housed the pathology and physiology departments of the B. J. Medical College at a nominal rent of 1 rupee per year.[56] The VRC was formally inaugurated by Kaur on February 4, 1953. Since the RF had a program for strengthening medical education in various key areas of India, it made efforts to tie the virus research laboratory operation with existing university facilities. In 1963, a program of graduate and postgraduate education was finalized with AIIMS.[57]

RF and ICMR Cooperation: Nature and Form

The VRC was designated as a cooperative project of the RF and the ICMR. The ICMR was handicapped by a lack of funds and trained personnel, while the RF's aid and assistance would be a great help to the development and consolidation of the work of ICMR, all existing medical colleges, and medical research and training institutions. The ICMR had a local fellowship training program with which the RF's foreign fellowship training program could be coordinated.

The RF, the ICMR and the Indian government agreed that the VRC was to be financed by the RF and a special appropriation of the Ministry of Health. Until the Centre was fully developed and able to function permanently, the RF was to be responsible for assigning specially trained senior scientific personnel and paying the salaries and travel expenses of these personnel. It was to provide the services of experts in virology and in entomology.[58] The RF specifically would send

> a small group, perhaps four, of our staff members experienced in various aspects of virus work to India to set up a well equipped virus laboratory which would serve as a center for the training of personnel and for the

investigation of virus diseases of importance in India. It would ... conduct epidemiological surveys to determine which virus diseases are prevalent and which ones appear to be of greatest interest.[59]

The RF staff would train Indians in all essential fields of virology. The RF would select promising local medical professionals and other personnel for specialized training, both locally and overseas, to develop individual skills and capabilities so that ultimately, they would assume responsibility for these laboratories. The RF was to establish standards of excellence for medical research in general, and to train local personnel in "many of the most important techniques necessary for modern work in the broad field of microbiology."[60] This would consist of techniques of virus isolation, their identification, entomological research, epidemiological research through field surveys and tissue culture methods. Additionally, the RF was asked to make a major contribution to the program by providing most of the permanent and expendable laboratory equipment, especially those which needed to be imported from abroad.

The ICMR was required to provide a suitable space for the central laboratory, a substantial contribution toward the maintenance of the laboratory and fieldwork and the purchase of expendable supplies and assign personnel—professional, technical and clerical—to the unit and pay their salaries.[61] Once the Indian staff was fully trained the RF personnel would be withdrawn on a mutually agreed date and the center would then be run as a full-fledged unit of the ICMR. The RF trustees underlined that the success of the laboratory would depend on it becoming "an integral and self-perpetuating part of the local research and public health effort."[62]

In September 1951, John Austin Kerr of the IHD was appointed as director of the VRC. He arrived in New Delhi in October 1951 to undertake the preliminary organization of the centre such as setting up the laboratories and recruiting the staff.[63] Kerr and Pandit agreed that the VRC was to develop into a permanent program either separately or as a part of some larger medical research institute.[64] Kerr insisted that the RF directorship of the VRC was not negotiable. He wrote to Robert Morison, director of the DMPH: "If things should get to such a state that an Indian were appointed as Director against our wishes, then would be the time we picked our marbles and went home."[65] His argument to Watson was: "After all, our major contribution consists of our technical knowledge of virus research, with the provision of dollars which are scarce, for the procurement of necessary equipment being rather secondary in importance."[66] Kerr was responsible for the overall administration, planning and implementation of the research aspects. Harald N. Johnson, a RF staff member, was given responsibility for the technical direction of laboratory procedures, including the training of personnel in these procedures. After Johnson left, other RF staff, zoologist Brooke Worth, virologist Telford H. Work and biologist Harold Trapido, joined the VRC. Work would later assume the directorship of the VRC from Kerr. The Indian staff consisted of

T. Ramachandra Rao, a medical entomologist; B.S. Lamba, an ornithologist; and research officers Keerti Shah, Pravin Bhatt and Khorshed Pavri.

The RF did not believe that one laboratory would suffice to study all the virus problems uncovered by the VRC. In addition to its own work, the centre could aid and stimulate virus studies of all sorts by other workers. In a letter to Lakshmanan, Warren suggested the RF would assist the development of a few virus units in other Indian research institutions. The RF would train personnel and assist with technical advice. It even showed a willingness to donate essential equipment.[67] Over the years, the VRC developed contacts with the virus laboratory of the Armed Forces Medical College in Poona, Christian Medical College in Vellore, the Poliomyelitis Research Unit of the ICMR, the Seth G.S. Medical College in Bombay, the Central Research Institute in Kasauli, the King Institute in Madras, the Central Drug Institute in Lucknow, the AllHPH and the Pasteur Institute in Coonoor.

In April 1955, the Scientific Advisory Board and governing body of the ICMR recommended that under the second Five-Year-Plan, the VRC be enlarged at the cost of Rs 1 million (approximately US$210,000) and converted into a Virus Research Institute, at which all virus research would be concentrated.[68] By 1957 the then VRC director, Work, claimed that the centre had established itself as "not only the primary institution of its kind in India but the most well developed virological facility between Cairo and Tokyo and Kuala Lumpur and Singapore."[69] The Indian government appropriated Rs. 450,000 for the building of a new wing to the existing laboratory. The new addition was expected to double the existing space and provide additional modern and suitable quarters for certain phases of the work. This expansion, however, required certain equipment and specialized apparatus from abroad. The RF was already supplying specialized personnel presently unavailable in India and had paid for the equipment and supplies that needed foreign exchange. With the new plans, the RF was asked to provide an additional $70,000 for equipping the new building.[70] The RF Trustees acceded to the request and made the necessary grant. From 1951 to 1964, the RF had given the VRC approximately $1,180,000.[71]

The VRC: Scope of Work

The VRC was organized for the study of filterable viruses affecting humans and their domestic animals. It was especially important for India, as it had a large rural population primarily engaged in agriculture. Special interest was in those viruses that were transmitted by bloodsucking arthropods. Epidemiological studies done in other places, especially in Africa and Latin America indicated that some of those viruses had a "reservoir" in small mammals and birds and that there was an overflow from that reservoir to man and to domestic animals such as horses. The researchers at the VRC would focus on these small warm-blooded vertebrates. The approach would be broadly ecological that would entail a great deal of fieldwork.[72] Underscoring the significance of their work, Kerr explained to K.V. Krishnan, Director of the AIIHPH:

> It is obvious that there are many undescribed viruses which infect man and his domestic animals; and it is equally obvious that viruses are the least well known of the micro-organisms which infect man and his domestic animals. We like to think that we are opening up the last frontier of microbiology.[73]

The goals of VRC were to define the distribution of arthropod-borne virus diseases in the various regions of India, collect and identify new viruses and study their natural history. It was to bring to the notice of authorities those viruses and their carriers that were important from the public health point of view and advise the government on appropriate control measures. Within five years of its establishment, four departments were set up at the VRC, namely, Virology, Field Epidemiology, Zoology and Entomology.

There was little knowledge about the prevalence of important virus diseases in India that were known to occur in different parts of the world. It was hoped that eventually many diseases in India would be identified with viruses. They could be some of those which the RF had already under observation among the fourteen odd "wild viruses" collected in Africa and South America.[74] The work and the efforts that followed could mean

> that within a short period of years a considerable volume of worthwhile information can be brought to light which will be of great significance to the future health of the Indians, as well as to the other countries of the world.[75]

The research involved importing into India the viruses collected and stored for reference at the RFVL against which the newly discovered VRC viruses were to be tested for both identification and immunity. RF officials, however, chose to exercise caution with respect to importing into India the viruses because they had no means of knowing whether these viruses or strains existed in India. As a precaution, therefore, it was proposed that the laboratory program in India "in the initial stages would probably have to consist of collection of sera for immunity tests in New York and the isolation of new virus strains."[76] Elaborating on the exploratory start to virus research in India, Kenneth Smithburn of the DMPH Laboratories postulated the presence of the Russian Spring Summer Encephalitis (RSSE) or Japanese B viruses in India on the ground that both were present in East Asia. Japanese B virus was also known to be present in the Pacific islands. Both RSSE and Japanese B were arthropod viruses but with different epidemiology according to existing knowledge. RSSE, was, however, more likely to be associated with jungle and bush regions than Japanese B. Smithburn suggested that the RF staff in India collect some sera for tests to be conducted in New York against these and other viruses prior to the establishment of virus investigations in India. "If it could be discovered that some virus which we already have is present and active in India, the individuals who are to be responsible for laboratory studies there would have a good jump-ing-off point."[77] The field studies carried out in India would be supplemented by laboratory studies. Until the laboratory in Poona was ready, they would undertake immunity tests while the sera thus collected would be shipped to New York.[78] This exercise was expected to give an idea of the spectrum of virus antibodies present in the country.

Under the direction of the RF, the VRC staff, in early 1952, commenced a reconnaissance of virus immunity of two particular virus diseases, namely, Jap-anese B and RSSE. The activity, however, provided wider results. By early 1954, a good number of viruses had been isolated from birds, mosquitoes, and mites in India. These preliminary finds "tend to substantiate the evidence obtained from the immunity survey that virus infections are highly prevalent in India."[79] Officials in the New York office, however, felt that the program had so far placed too much emphasis on studies of birds, arthropods and mammals and that it was time to direct the field studies more toward humans. "The dif-ficulty," as Smith wrote to Kerr, "is to find out maybe the significance of these newly isolated viruses as etiological agents of human and animal disease. It will undoubtedly require much intensive study to establish these points."[80] Kerr initiated the collection of human sera for immunity tests in the Devimane area of Kanara district and villages of Manjari and Baramati near Poona.

The VRC also served as a public health laboratory for the government at different times to tackle outbreaks of epidemic diseases. At the request and insistence of the ICMR and the Ministry of Health, the VRC conducted inves-tigations into six different epidemics notably the Jamshedpur fever, Vellore fever, hepatitis in Delhi and the Kyasanur forest disease (KFD) that broke out between 1954 and 1962. A considerable deal of time and resources at the VRC was diverted toward investigations into the epidemics. The KFD is a good example to illustrate the work.

KFD: Research and Vaccine Production in India

A new epidemic broke out in the Kysanaur forest in the Shimoga district of Mysore (present-day Karnataka) state in March 1957. The staff at VRC received reports that villages were suffering from a severe and unusual disease and that monkeys were dying in large numbers in the surrounding forest areas. The VRC formed a team to visit the area led by Work and Trapido. With the sup-port of a field group that was engaged in the epidemiological study of enceph-alitis in the Vellore area, the VRC directed a major portion of facilities and staff toward the elucidation of what later came to be named KFD. The RFVL as was the practice was involved in these investigations as well.

Within three weeks of its arrival, the VRC team had isolated the virus strains from both humans and monkeys who were suffering a prolonged and prostrat-ing febrile illness, which caused a substantial number of human fatalities. The viruses found in humans and monkeys were identical, and the recovered patients had developed antibodies to the isolated agent. Tests identified the isolated virus as being very similar to the virus of RSSE and Omsk hemorrhagic fever. The virus was also isolated from a series of ticks and thus appeared to be tick-borne. Public health records of the region suggested that a few cases of the disease had probably occurred in the same area in 1956 but not before. During the spring and summer of 1957, the disease appeared to have spread rapidly through the forest and the minimum area involved was approximately 500 square miles. By winter, approximately 500 people were thought to have been infected, and about 50 of them died. There appeared some hope of containing further spread by intensive control measures directed at the local tick population and the monkey (and presumably rodent) reservoir in the area.[81] As a result, efforts were undertaken to determine the forest cycle and the rate of spread of the disease.[82]

By early 1959, the VRC had established a well-equipped field station to track the progress of KFD in Mysore. The VRC-led investigations suggested that KFD was present in certain areas of Mysore for some time and that the epidemic outbreak in 1957 probably represented a flare-up of preexisting infection rather than a new introduction. Although vaccination with an RSSE vaccine proved to have inadequate protection, the number of human cases declined in both 1958 and 1959. Early identification and treatment of cases appeared to have reduced the death rate.[83]

The investigations by the VRC team also made a significant discovery: it "turned up a good deal of evidence that throws doubt upon a long-held Russian hypothesis that the passage of virus from adult to larval ticks is an important element in the maintenance of the tick-borne viruses in nature."[84] Immunological surveys conducted there "tended to play down the role of small rodents and enhance that of large domestic species as carriers of KFD."[85] The VRC established a systematic monitoring system to gain more precise knowledge of the ebb and flow of the virus activity, accompanied by intensive studies of the basic questions about the epidemiology of KFD.[86] The preliminary work in Shimoga indicated that Japanese B encephalitis had followed a similar pattern, but further observation and careful investigation were required before any definite answers about its epidemiology could be found.[87] By 1964, the VRC had completed the first phase of its investigations of identifying the agents and the vectors of the disease. The second phase began in 1965 to define the natural cycle of KFD and unravel the mystery surrounding the peculiar behavior of these agents in human beings.[88]

As deaths associated with the KFD continued to rise, a vaccination program was conducted in the area. The initial tests had shown similarities between KFD and RSSE, and health officials decided to use an RSSE vaccine. In April 1956, the Indian government imported 3,000 doses of the RSSE vaccine from Moscow. It took the ICMR one month to obtain a translation of the Russian instructions, but even after one year had passed, the vaccine had neither been tested nor used. They continued to rest in the refrigerator of the Chest

Institute. Work, on his own initiative, decided to test the vaccine in Poona. But M.C. Balfour, resident director for the RF in New Delhi, observed that the Russian vaccine's "intentions and performance are not the same in India."[89] Work noted "that the problem has been uncovered and that the further dealing with it as a disease in people is the responsibility of the medical and public health authorities of Mysore State."[90]

At the end of August 1957, the director general of health services called a conference on KFD in Bangalore (now Bengaluru).[91] Another conference was followed on September 4, 1957, in the office of the Central Minister of Health, D.P. Karmarkar, who had been elected a member of parliament from Mysore state. It was attended by the health secretary; three members of parliament from Mysore; three members of Indian Army Medical Corps; General Rao, D.M.S., a representative from the AIIHPH; and a medical consultant, Col. Naik, apart from Pandit, Balfour and Work. Work made his presentation stressing the rapid spread of the disease. Naik, who discussed the clinical aspects of the cases with reference to the RSSE, argued that since eradication was impracticable, the production of a vaccine was recommended. Work felt that given the severity of the disease, the authorities could not wait until a vaccine was produced in Indian facilities and hence emphasized the urgency of conducting vaccination immediately. It was decided to bring the supply of RSSE vaccine from American sources that could be made available immediately. The vaccine was imported from the army laboratory at the Walter Reed Hospital in Washington, D.C., in small batches. Arrangements were made to manufacture enough vaccine to protect the 50,000 people most likely to be exposed to the disease. It was proposed that India was to develop the production of vaccine after dealing with the initial emergency.[92]

When the vaccination campaign was decided, Balfour had noted that such a campaign would require planning and preparation. In particular, he considered it essential to place a competent and effective person in full charge of the program, but the health authorities had failed to even discuss the matter.[93] Balfour's concerns were justified when some of the staff involved in the campaign were infected with the vaccine and the vaccination had to be discontinued. However, the Ministry of Health expressed the desire to continue the vaccination campaign and requested the RF to supply an additional 50,000 doses of RSSE vaccine.[94] Work pointed out that 10,000 doses had been dispatched, on the request from the chief secretary of Mysore, and were in use in Shimoga. He assured the ministry that further stock was available for immediate delivery.[95]

The vaccine from Walter Reed Hospital of Washington, D.C., was prepared through a formalinized suspension of mouse brain, which was quite expensive to manufacture and uncertain in its effects. It was, therefore, proposed to develop an attenuated living vaccine similar to the vaccine against smallpox and yellow fever. This would be a long-term effort. The work of developing modern tissue culture in both the Poona and New York laboratories was carried out because the staff had been prepared to undertake the investigation.[96] Another problem with the vaccine being imported from the US was that it was prepared by inactivating RSSE with formalin. RSSE was used because it was the best-known agent in the group of diseases, which included KFD. But KFD itself proved somewhat difficult to handle under production conditions. With the help of the staff at the Walter Reed laboratory, who undertook intensive research to find a more effective preparation, a suitable KFD strain was made available to produce a vaccine in India by the end of 1958. Some of the Indian staff from the VRC participated actively in the work at the Walter Reed laboratory and received training to undertake local production in India.[97]

In order to prepare for possibly more severe epidemics in the future a small unit for the experimental production of a more suitable vaccine was set up in the Haffkine Institute with staff provided by the VRC.[98] Keerti Shah of the VRC was put in charge to supervise the production, with C.N. Dandawate as a research assistant. The progress of vaccine production at the Haffkine Institute was slow primarily because of red tape and the bureaucratic functioning of the relevant government departments and the Ministry of Health. The original estimates made by the Public Works Department of the government of Bombay to remodel the laboratory were found to be too low and the subsequent calculations and approval took a long time. Similar experiences happened to the import of equipment for vaccine production from abroad, which was partially financed by the RF.[99]

The ICMR made grants for the import of equipment, but India faced a foreign exchange crisis during this period. The ICMR was required to obtain permission from the government, which it did not receive until January 1960.[100] The ICMR also applied for an import license from the government to import equipment. By the time the license permit arrived, the grant had expired. The ICMR had to reapply for the grant. Charles. R. Anderson, who had replaced Work as director of VRC, was apparently frustrated and observed that "it would appear that by the time the grant is renewed, the import permit will expire, so that things seem to be going in an unfortunate circle."[101]

Regarding the ongoing vaccine problem, there was frustration about the research itself. Morison felt that there was a need for rethinking. He wrote to Anderson:

> it seems to me it is probably not very wise to devote one's energies to the development of an inactivated mouse brain preparation for general use. Everybody who has tried it has become discouraged, and for very good reasons. The alternatives would seem to be an inactivated tissue culture in egg preparation or an attenuated strain.

He further added, "Unless KFD develops into a more serious and immediate public health hazard than it as now, I would tend to vote for concentration in the attenuated strain since I am sure this will be the only satisfactory long-term solutions."[102] Anderson concurred with Morison about the mouse brain vaccine and pointed out that part of the program was to investigate the possibility of chick embryos. Anderson himself was working on the attenuated problem.[103] The reason for undertaking the inactivated or killed vaccine preparation was because Pandit had favored the approach. Neither Anderson nor Morison agreed with him, and the former had conveyed this to Pandit. Both, however, realized they had little choice but to comply because the decision had been made by Pandit himself as head of the ICMR.[104]

Viruses and Migratory Birds

The VRC investigations noted that the KFD virus was closely related to the Omsk hemorrhagic fever and the RSSE, suggesting that the viruses might have arrived in India through migratory birds that flew in every September and October from Russia and Siberia to Kutch and Saurashtra regions of Gujarat. Furthermore, an antibody survey in 1952 in Saurashtra had indicated that a member of the RSSE virus could be active in India. This was confirmed in January 1958 by human serum collection in the area.[105] Work was keen that the VRC undertake further research into this. Salim Ali, India's foremost ornithologist and head of the Bombay Natural History Society (BNHS) had undertaken bird ringing or banding to study migratory birds since the 1930s. Later Ali proposed the setting up of a series of migratory bird-observation stations in Kutch and carrying out bird banding. Work saw in this an opportunity for the VRC.

He explained to Rusk why and how such research was necessary: that ornithologists had little to no interest in the matter but virologists globally who until then had confined their research to laboratories had begun to show an increasing interest in investigating migratory birds transporting viruses across geographical areas and national boundaries; India offered a rare opportunity given that Kutch and Saurashtra witnessed bird migration apart from Russia from eastern China and South Africa across land and sea routes; and the thaw in relations with the Soviets had opened possibilities of cooperation with Soviet scientists that was recognized both in the US and India.[106]

The idea that this investigation could be undertaken with Soviet cooperation was significant for both Soviet and American scientists had recognized and initiated steps towards public health and medical research notwithstanding the Cold War as seen earlier. The easing of relations between the US and the USSR made such an eventuality further likely and practical. It was suggested that the Soviets could undertake banding of specific species in their region some of whom flew to India. The Soviets could also exchange information about viruses, ticks and birds. And as Work noted, "If they (birds) contained antibodies, virus, similar ticks or ticks infected with virus, we should have established for the first time through such a joint effort the importance of migratory birds as long-distance vectors of arbor virus."[107] They could also examine the same birds or those marked by Indians when they returned to Russia during summer and examine them for ticks and viruses that were probably transported from the tropics such as India.

Work suggested that the RF approach Anatoli A. Smoridentsev, chief of the Virus Research Laboratories of the All Union Institute of Experimental Medicine in Leningrad, an authority on RSSE virus, and Mikhail. P. Chumakov, mentioned earlier with reference to polio, of the Institute of Neurology of the Academy of Medical Sciences in Moscow, an authority on RSS hemorrhagic fever virus, who were going to be present at the Lisbon meetings of the International Congress for Tropical Medicine. Instead of Russian ornithologists, these two were likely to have more influence in the Russian Academy of Sciences, the sanctioning authority for such cooperation and which, in 1955, had become a member of the International Science Council. If they were disposed to such cooperation, then India might sponsor an official proposition for Indians had shown an inclination for such cooperative studies and had all the potential for such investigations. Most important, India was nonaligned. Furthermore, Work noted,

> Beyond the potential scientific accomplishments, this sort of exploration of international cooperation with Russia by a private organization such as ours might be highly significant in a much broader way and serve as an example for other such cooperative scientific biological investigations which you (Rusk) have proposed.[108]

Work went on to add, "It is merely what seems to me a practical proposition implementing a suggestion you have publicly pronounced as a basis for cooperation in man's fight with nature."[109]

Later in May 1960, Smoridentsev, who was a short-term consultant to the WHO in Cairo, at the request of the WHO to India's Ministry of Health, visited India and the VRC. Smoridentsev had already got the Soviet Ministry of Health to write to Rusk in February 1960 for a "free exchange" between the scientists of the USSR and those of the RF.[110] In Poona, in his discussion with Trapido, he spoke of the desirability of a Central World Reference Laboratory for the arbor viruses and expressed the view that India was the most appropriate place to have this laboratory. He delineated the reasons (1) India's nonalignment made it possible for scientists across the world to come there, (2) the presence of the already-RF-supported VRC, and (3) India as a region had myriad virus problems that were immediately available and accessible for investigation. Anderson and Trapido were noncommittal about the idea, although Smoridentsev persisted and pushed the idea, especially since he believed the VRC staff had the experience and competence apart from the financial support of the RF while WHO participation was indicated because of its supranational position.[111] This idea, for reasons buried in archival documents, however, did not materialize.

Trapido, who had evinced interest in the BNHS bird banding project in Kutch, discussed with Salim Ali the possibilities of conducting virus research among these migratory birds which stimulated much interest in the society's members. The BNHS at the time was under consideration for a significant grant from the RF to develop its facilities, and hence, it could be expected to take an interest in the VRC research concerns, which were primarily serological and ectoparasite collections.[112]

The BNHS had been unable to raise funds for the Kutch study, but with the outbreak of the KFD and the interest expressed by Trapido, Ali claimed to have found an unsolicited opportunity. He observed: "The apparently transcontinental distribution of the virus suggested it could have reached here through the agency of ticks on birds migrating between USSR and India."[113]

For the WHO, this required serious and immediate attention. Dr A.C. Saenz, who was in charge of virus diseases in the Division of Communicable Diseases at the WHO, called a meeting of "Scientific Group on Research on Birds as Disseminators of Arthropod-borne Viruses" in March 1959 in Geneva, and Ali was invited to attend. At the meeting, Ali was asked to prepare a project proposal for the study of bird migration in northwest India that would cover an examination of how birds carried arbor viruses. The proposal titled "Studies on Birds as Possible Disseminators of Arthropod Borne Viruses" was approved. In so titling it, Ali suggested to the RF officers at VRC an "*a priori* joint project between the VRC and BNHS." Anderson and Trapido were uneasy about this, and the latter informed Ali that the project be renamed so that it would not in any way imply VRC participation as integral to the BNHS investigation.[114] Trapido simultaneously made a similar request to Saenz to exclude any suggestion of direct VRC involvement in the project. He made it clear to Saenz that VRC, given other commitments, would examine the birds only for ticks and not store or study sera.[115] Saenz not too happy proposed some limited participation since a purely ornithological study would be difficult to justify to the division at the WHO.[116] RF officials acknowledged that WHO would be reluctant to give funds for a project that did not include the study of viruses.

Funds were not available from the WHO medical research program, but US$1000 were sanctioned from the WHO regular budget to the BNHS given the importance of the study and in expectation that supplementary money could be obtained from the Indian Government or other institutes.[117] Ali sought additional funds from the RF and requested from the VRC a definite commitment for cooperation.[118] Pandit had already indicated to Trapido that any expansion of VRC activities beyond those in operation would require prior permission of the ICMR. Pandit probably had reservations with any VRC engagement with the BNHS project since this was being carried out in areas close to the Pakistan border and hence had a bearing on defense and national security matters.[119] As seen earlier, relations between the USA and India were by this time already tense and testy. It seemed ICMR was unlikely to grant permission for any such cooperation between the VRC and BNHS. Trapido informed Pandit that Anderson and he agreed that VRC participation could be limited to studying the kinds and frequency of ectoparasites or ticks in migratory birds and not conduct sera studies that could also place a burden on the ongoing work at the VRC. RF officials in New York agreed to such limited participation with clearance from the ICMR.[120]

In 1960 the BNHS received funds from the WHO."[121] By this time, RF officials admitted that KFD appeared unlikely or was only remotely connected with any viruses found beyond the Himalayas. Morison further noted that there appeared little reason to divert VRC resources to the "bird business" merely because of global pressure to undertake such studies.[122] By mid-1960s, KFD also subsided without spreading to other regions. Four years later, the funding to the BNHS ceased as the WHO was forced to curb its contribution to various public health and research programs.

Funds, however, came from the Smithsonian Institution and the Migratory Animals Pathological Survey (MAPS) program, which was undertaken by the US Army Medical Research Laboratory and funded by US Army Research and Development Group (Far East). MAPS was a bigger bird-ringing project covering five countries in Southeast Asia and was directed to investigate Japanese encephalitis, among other infectious diseases.[123] The funding, however, stipulated that Ali share data and samples with MAPS. Interestingly, Soviet scientists were also involved with Ali's project. Ali, with MAPS approval, visited the USSR to share his data and samples with the Soviets. Nithyanand Rao notes: "Despite that, a controversy erupted over the American army funding the project with possible eye on biological weapons. Knowing bird migrations routes, critics felt, could open the door to their usage for the delivery of viruses across international borders."[124] Ali ascribed the controversy to an alarmist newspaper report that suggested that the BNHS was working in collusion with the US "to explore the possibility of migratory birds being used in biological warfare for inducting and disseminating deadly viruses and germs in enemy countries." Since Indian migrant birds came from the USSR, and possibly also China, this lent credibility to the report in view of the Cold War, which had heated up considerably about this time. The report caused an uproar in government and political quarters in Delhi. It "generated much heat and voice among our pro-Communist, anti-US patriots in the Lok Sabha."[125]

Part of the controversy also appears to have arisen from the fact that Dillon Ripley, an ecologist and Yale professor, was Ali's partner in the bird banding project. Ripley had been chief of the Office of Strategic Services (OSS) secret service branch in Southeast Asia during WWII. The OSS was the forerunner of the CIA, and even though Ripley was no longer associated with it, doubts remained.[126] Michael Lewis, who has written a detailed account of this episode, comments that it

> confirmed fears of those Indians who suspected that US scientists such as Ripley, who kept requesting permission to walk around in sensitive border areas like the forests along the border of India, China or Nepal, were collecting information that was not always strictly ornithological. What better cover could a secret agent ask for than to be an ecologist of remote species or ecosystems?[127]

Michael Lewis, in referring to ecologists, in particular, and scientists, in general, observes that many of them during this period acted "as if their research funding did not have any political or ethical import."[128]

Criticism of and Allegations against the VRC

However, as seen, the VRC was not directly involved with the BNHS project when the controversy involving the latter broke out, but it raised questions and suspicions about the VRC and its work. The VRC had always been viewed with suspicion by many sections within the government, the parliament, the medical profession and the public. Soon after the VRC was established, "a high government official at a cabinet meeting stated he believed that the purpose of the RF in establishing the laboratory was to do research in bacteriological warfare and then pass on the information to the Germans." This was apparently reported by Kaur to an RF official while explaining how in India open suspicion of the RF's motives was voiced not infrequently even in high places.[129]

Other questions were raised in the parliament, where aspersions were cast on the objectives and nature of the work of the VRC. Reports and articles in party papers and journals commented on the need to closely monitor the VRC and demanded tighter government control of it. For instance, in March 1953, Dr. R. B. Gour asked in the parliament if the government of India had control over the VRC and if foreigners working at the institute used it for purposes of developing germ warfare. The deputy minister for health, Smt. Chandrashekhar, replied that the VRC was a collaboration between the Indian government and the RF and that it conducted research into virus diseases particular to India.[130] This was an unsatisfactory answer as members of parliament continued to ask questions.

Ironically, Sokhey, then a member of the Council of States or the upper house of the Indian Parliament, raised serious objections about the functioning of VRC and the role of the RF. As stated earlier, Sokhey was among the former RF fellows and the senior Indian officials whom the RF officials had consulted prior to the establishment of VRC and counted on to extend support to the VRC. Archival sources indicate mutual respect between Sokhey and the RF. It is, therefore, unclear what his motives were. Sokhey was known to have Communist sympathies. It is probable that Sokhey's target was Pandit, suggesting professional differences or jealousies. If Kerr is to be believed, "Pandit was under some pressure to justify the considerable sum being spent by the ICMR on the VRC, largely because of needling by Major General Sokhey who is now a member of the Council of States."[131] Kerr received a letter from ICMR asking for details of ICMR and RF expenses so that a question in Parliament could be answered.[132] The questions were "presumably on the basis that the ICMR is wasting money by financing pure research at the VRC."[133] For Kerr, this meant that "the sooner the VRC can present some concrete results, the better off it will be."[134]

Sokhey did not appear to have relented and persisted in asking more questions in subsequent sessions of parliament. There were "vague allegations" of espionage by the American director and about germ warfare. To counter these allegations and suspicions, Pandit made vigorous efforts to defend the VRC. Scientific publicity about the work of the VRC was suggested, apart from which Pandit had Kerr prepare a long memorandum on the activities of the VRC to be submitted to Kaur and Nehru who was equally interested in the VRC work. Kaur was expected to use the information to prepare a comprehensive reply to the questions.[135]

The questions which had been submitted in advance as per procedure were never asked, for it appeared that they were disallowed by the chairman of the House under the advice of Nehru. The questions—not in exactly those words— were along these lines:

> Is it true that The Rockefeller Foundation is supporting a laboratory for Virus Research in Poona? At what address? Are the two American Doctors, J.A. Kerr and H.N. Johnson, in charge of the work? Is it true that the virus (or germs) of yellow fever are used in this laboratory? Is it true that insects and small animals are infected with the viruses? Is it true that these researches are not concerned with the curing of disease?[136]

The questions were "presumably Communist-inspired," and Sokhey was suspected to be responsible for them.[137]

The suspicion about "Communist-inspired" questions received a fillip when the *New Age Weekly*, a journal of the Communist Party of India, published a report in April 1955 titled "Fishy U.S.–Directed Virus Research Programme." The report claimed that "[s]urprise is expressed in medical circles here about the strange way in which research is being conducted at the Virus Research Centre." It further maintained that though the amount budgeted for the VRC was far more than the combined total for all such projects of the ICMR, it did not conduct any research in virus strains that were isolated but simply shipped them to the New York laboratories for study there. The other charges were that the VRC was conducting research not in infectious diseases widely prevalent in India, such as smallpox or influenza, but hunting insect-borne viruses in which the RF was interested. Moreover, with only one American director and one very junior worker to assist him, and the rest merely technical personnel and menials, "the centre cannot but remain just a field unit for purposes which will remain known to the American centre alone."[138]

The final allegation was the VRC's engagement in the development of some kind of biological weapons. This suspicion was elaborated, suggesting that the insect-borne viruses being studied at the VRC were common among wild birds and mammals that produced severe epidemic diseases like yellow fever or encephalitis. The report acknowledged that yellow fever might not be a threat to India since it was a well-established fact that it did not exist in India but expressed fear that if a virus with yellow fever trait was developed with another trait found in parasites in some wild birds and with similar high infectivity to humans, then "it would be possible in course of time to produce a mixed strain having a double potentiality for both man and bird. Such a strain will carry epidemic to men while not causing the same to birds." The report went on to argue that such a laboratory-based mutation virulent to humans and wildlife alike and as deadly as yellow fever was possible in an institution that collected and maintained an international pool of insect-borne viruses. It pointed out that the RFVL in New York was such a center. In addition, the *New Age Weekly* stated that some American virologists were of the opinion that such a mutant had the potential "for creating an epidemic because the wild animals or birds carrying the virus would remain living. Besides, the irregular picture of the epidemic would elude effective control at least for some time causing terrible devastation." More important, the *New Age Weekly* further suggested that the work conducted at the VRC was opaque. It appeared to lack transparency, observing,

> In view of the strange manner of work at the Poona Centre, medical circles are asking: What was there to prevent it from being utilised as an adjunct for some such purpose as surmised above? ... without any access into the doings of the New York institution it is not possible to confirm or reject them.

The reason for the suspicions was due to "the diabolical record of American germ warfare in China and Korea." The *New Age Weekly* called on the government of India to "investigate into the matter and, at any rate, to insist that virus research be conducted at the Poona Station for Indian needs instead of being a field appendage of the American centre."[139]

The same allegations were repeated in May 1955 in *Yugantar*, a Marathi weekly, published from Poona with communist leanings. In a letter to Dr. B.B. Dikshit, the Surgeon General of Bombay, who later became the first director of the All India Institute of Medical Sciences in Delhi, Work asserted:

> The absurdity of the contents are [*sic*] hardly worth notice. Surgeon General is well acquainted with our activity and was instrumental in establishing the VRC. ... Our activities are widely publicized through our Annual Reports, papers published in scientific journals and in reports published by the ICMR. The Americans working in this institution are here at the express invitation of the Central Government of India and we feel sure that this invitation would not be extended if the activities of such officers were in question.[140]

Suspicion about and allegations against the VRC and its American association would continue well into the late 1960s.

Concluding Remarks

The influence and impact of the RF's virus program were felt worldwide. The late 1950s saw a considerable growth of interest in the importance of arthropod-borne animal viruses. The epidemiological branch of the WHO organized several informal conferences on the subject. The RF's training program served to strengthen ties with many outside laboratories. By the 1960s, a inter-laboratory flow of personnel, information and materials had developed.[141]

It was in this broad context that this chapter examined the foreign and international aid to India's virus research and preventive medicine program during the early years of the Cold War. It focused on the RF's virus research program and how it laid the foundation of virology research in India. It discussed the reasons and purposes of the program, which was but a part of the RF's global plan for virus research. India was able to build up knowledge of viruses through the studies at the VRC and used the knowledge to address some of the epidemics that broke out during this period. Suspicions about the VRC work were influenced by anti-American sentiments that were generated by the Cold War politics and certain aspects of American foreign policy. The criticism and allegations directed against the VRC clearly reflected the misgivings and distrust about the US, in general, and the RF, in particular. This chapter illuminates that certain responses to domestic and foreign policies and wariness about the activities of foreign actors, especially if these were perceived adverse to national interest, were natural within the particular international environment of that era. Global health requires that international cooperation and collaboration be encouraged to advance medical science and its benefits to humankind.

Internationalization, politicization and militarization have very clearly made medical or virus research a contested and contentious area and have created doubts in the minds of large sections of the population about both curative and preventive health care systems. Medical history has shown us that through the ages in wars and battles, various infectious diseases have killed more soldiers than the fighting itself. Gradually, the possibilities of decimating rival forces through the deliberate action of spreading disease among the enemy were realized. Medical and especially virology research thus had two major aspects: not only protecting the health of people but also developing biological weapons to annihilate enemies. This has been particularly the case in the twentieth century as nuclear weapons used only once have become mainly weapons of deterrence than war, despite threats from those having nuclear weapons. An alternative has been the research and development of biological weapons. This has added suspicions about genuine medical research that has helped to overcome and even eradicate some dreadful diseases to reduce mortality rates and increase life expectancy.

Virology research is an important component of public health and preventive medicine. Virus research has both therapeutic and prophylactic benefits. Virology research has also been at the center of conspiratorial theories, fearmongering, rumors and controversies of various kinds. Unethical practices by pharmaceutical companies, medical laboratories and medical research, biological warfare laboratories are realities that cannot be brushed aside. Questions have been raised about the "celebrity philanthropy" and philanthro-capitalism, some being indeed of concern.[142] They are part of our reality. Some conspiracies have origins in delusions and deranged minds while some are deliberate and planned actions. Both are part of our reality and matters of concern.

There is another reality. The reality of the WHO, UNICEF, Red Cross, Doctors without Borders and what Anne-Emanuelle Birn and Theodore M Brown refer to as "Comrades in Health" that form the pillars of global health.[143] The One Health concept formulated in 2004 that draws from the One Medicine concept advocated by Calvin Schwabe approaches the linkage between humans, animals and the environment to understand and explain health and medical care.[144] The IHR (2005) and the Global Health Security Agenda embarked on in 2014 are action-oriented programs that seek to enhance and encourage participation, coordination and collaboration among countries and other multiple stakeholders to deal with health threats from emerging and reemerging infectious diseases. International cooperation and collaboration in medical research are a necessity, but its politicization, militarization and conspiracy-mongering are what we need to be cautious and wary about.

Acknowledgments

Thanks are due to Corinna R. Unger, David Engerman, Anne-Emanuelle Birn, Robert Smith, Mangesh Kulkarni, Vivek Neelakantan and Dr. Mohan B. Dikshit for sharing or procuring reprints and photocopies of articles and sending copies of books and photographs. The chapter draws on two projects for which research and travel grants were received from the Rockefeller Foundation, Rockefeller Archive Center, the Sir Dorabji Tata Trust and the Wellcome Trust. Most important, my gratitude to Liping Bu for her consideration, patience and encouragement when the writing got tough with several health issues that plagued me during the period of writing.

Abbreviations

AIIHPH	All India Institute of Hygiene and Public Health
BNHS	Bombay Natural History Society
DMPH	Division of Medicine and Public Health
ICMR	Indian Council of Medical Research
IHR	International Health Regulations
KFD	Kysanaur Forest Disease
NIV	National Institute of Virology
RAC	Rockefeller Archive Center (all archives are from RAC unless otherwise specified)

RF	Rockefeller Foundation
RFVL	RF Virus Laboratory
RSSE	Russian Spring Summer Encephalitis
VRC	Virus Research Centre
WHO	World Health Organization

Notes

1 Vijay Kumar Chattu and W. Andy Knight, "Global Health Diplomacy as a Tool of Peace," *Peace Review* 32 (2019): 148–157, https://doi.org/10.1080/10402659.2019,1667563.
2 Ashish Bose, "Health Policy in India," in *Policy Making in India*, ed. K. D. Madan (New Delhi, Government of India, 1982): 501–519; Roger Jeffery, *The Politics of Health in India* (Berkeley, University of California Press, 1988); C. G. Pandit, *My World of Preventive Medicine, Indian Council of Medical Research, New Delhi* (1995); Sunil Amrith, "Political Culture of Health in India: A Historical Perspective," *Economic and Political Weekly* 42 (2007): 114–121.
3 Sunil Amrith, *Decolonizing International Health: South and Southeast Asia, 1930–65* (Basingstoke and New York, Palgrave Macmillan, 2006).
4 David Arnold, "Nehruvian Science and Postcolonial India," *Isis* 104 (2013): 360–370.
5 Ibid.
6 Ibid.
7 Shirish N. Kavadi, "Medicine, Philanthropy and Nationhood: Tensions of Different Visions in India," in *Public Health and National Reconstruction in Post-War Asia: International Influences, Local Transformations*, eds. Liping Bu and Ka-Che Yip (London and New York, Routledge, 2015): 132–153.
8 John A. Logan, "Counteracting Communism Through Foreign Assistance Programs in Public Health," *American Journal of Public Health* 45 (1955): 1017–1021; see also Chester Bowles, *Ambassador's Report* (New York, Harper and Brothers, 1954).
9 Marcos Cueto, "International Health, the Early Cold War and Latin America," *Canadian Bulletin of Medical History* 25 (2008): 17–41.
10 Ibid.
11 Theodore M. Brown, Marcos Cueto and Elizabeth Fee, "The World Health Organization: The Transition from 'International' to 'Global' Public Health," *American Journal of Public Health* 96 (2006): 62–72.
12 Gary R. Hess, "The Role of American Philanthropic Foundations in India's Road to Globalization during the Cold War Era," in *Globalization, Philanthropy, and Civil Society: Towards a New Political Culture in the Twenty-First Century*, eds. Soma Hewa and Darwin Stapleton (New York, Springer, 2006), 51–71.
13 Amrith, *Decolonizing International Health*; Jeffery, *The Politics of Health in India*.
14 M. I. Porras and M. J. Baguena, "The Role of the World Health Organization's Country Programs in the Development of Virology in Spain, 1951–1975," *Historia, Ciencias, Saude- Manguinhos* 27, Supplement (2020): 187–210.
15 Cueto, "International Health."
16 Ibid.
17 Ibid.
18 Tim Adams, book review of Epidemics and Society by Frank M. Snowden, *The Guardian Sun* May 10, 2020, https://www.theguardian.com/books/2020/may/10/epidemics-and-society-by-frank-m-snowden-review-illuminating-and-persuasiv.

19 Ibid.

20 Ibid.

21 Chattu and Knight, *Global Health Diplomacy.*

22 Erez Manela, "A Pox on Your Narrative: Writing Disease Control into Cold War History," *Diplomatic History* 34 (2010): 299–323, 300.

23 Chattu and Knight, *Global Health Diplomacy.* For a detailed account, see Saul Benison, "International Medical Cooperation: Dr. Albert Sabin, Live Poliovirus Vaccine and the Soviets," *Bulletin of the History of Medicine* 56 (1982): 460–483.

24 Bhore was an Indian Christian, born in present-day Maharashtra and educated at Bishop's School and Deccan College in Pune and subsequently in Britain. He was not British as is generally believed but had a British wife.

25 Kavadi, "Medicine, Philanthropy and Nationhood"; Jeffery, *The Politics of Health in India.*

26 Manu Bhagavan, ed., *India and the Cold War* (Gurugram, Penguin Random House India, 2019).

27 Amrith, *Decolonizing International Health.*

28 David C. Engerman, *The Price of Aid. The Economic Cold War in India* (Cambridge, MA, Harvard University Press, 2018), 3.

29 Jeffery, *The Politics of Health in India,* 246.

30 Kavadi, "Medicine, Philanthropy and Nationhood"; Jeffery, *The Politics of Health in India*; Leonard A. Gordon, "Wealth Equals Wisdom? The Rockefeller and Ford Foundations in India," *Annals of the American Academy of Political and Social Science* 554 (1997): 104–116.

31 Ross Bassett, *The Technological Indian* (Cambridge, MA, Harvard University Press, 2016); Kavadi, "Medicine, Philanthropy and Nationhood"; Gordon, "Wealth Equals Wisdom?"

32 See Kavadi, "The Cold War, Non-Alignment and Medicine in India: Medical Education and Pharmaceutical Self Sufficiency 1947–1957," in *The Geopolitics of Health in South and South East Asia: Perspectives from the Cold War to COVID-19, 1948–2021,* ed. Vivek Neelkantan (London and New York, Routledge, 2023); Nasir Tyabji, "Negotiating Nonalignment Dilemmas Attendant on Initiating Pharmaceutical Production in India," *Technology and Culture* 53 (2012): 37–60.

33 Vijay Singh, "Some strategies of Indian communists after 1947," in *India in the World since 1947: National and Transnational Perspectives,* eds. Andreas Hilger and Corinna R. Unger (Frankfurt, Peter Lang, 2012), 99–119; Swapna Kona Nayudu, "The Soviet Peace Offensive and Nehru's India, 1953–1956," in *India and the Cold War,* ed. Manu Bhagavan (Gurugram, Penguin Random House India, 2019): 36–56.

34 Tyabji, "Negotiating Nonalignment Dilemmas."

35 Andreas Hilger, "Building a Socialist Elite? – Khrushchev's Soviet Union and Elite Formation in India," in *Elites and Decolonization in the Twentieth Century,* eds. Jost Dulffer and Marc Frey (Basingstoke, Palgrave Macmillan, 2011): 262–286.

36 Kavadi, "Medicine, Philanthropy and Nationhood"; Kavadi, "The Cold War, Non-Alignment and Medicine in India."

37 Shirish N. Kavadi, *Rockefeller Foundation and Public Health in Colonial India, 1916–1945. A Narrative History,* The Foundation for Research in Community Health (Mumbai/Pune, 1999); "Rockefeller Public Health in Colonial India," in *Histories of Medicine and Healing in the Indian Ocean World, vol. 2,* eds. Anna Winterbottom and Facil Tesfaye (Basingstoke and New York, Palgrave Macmillan, 2016): 61–88; "Medicine, Philanthropy and Nationhood."

38 RF Board of Trustees Resolution, December 3–4, 1957; RG 1.2, S 464, Box 95, F 900, RAC. Also see Robert Shaplen, *Toward the Well-Being of Mankind. Fifty Years of The Rockefeller Foundation* (New York, Doubleday and Company, Inc, 1964).

39 Shaplen, *Toward the Well-Being of Mankind*, 44. Also, for a detailed account, see Wilbur G. Downs, "The Rockefeller Foundation Virus Program: 1951–1971 with Update to 1981," *Annual Review of Medicine* 33 (1982): 1–29. Downloaded from www.annualreviews.org.

40 RF Board of Trustees Resolution, December 3–4, 1957; RG 1.2, S 464, Box 95, F 900; Shaplen, *Toward The Well-Being of Mankind*.

41 RF Board of Trustees Resolution, December 4–5, 1951; RG 1.2, S 464 Box 95, F 900.

42 Shaplen, *Toward the Well-Being of Mankind*, 49.

43 The Indian Fund Research Fund Association was set up in 1911 to support medical research. In 1948, Pandit was invited by Kaur to become its first Indian secretary. It was redesignated as the Indian Council of Medical Research in 1949. Pandit later in the 1950s became its director.

44 Pandit, *My World*, 244.

45 Ibid., 245.

46 Watson to J. W. McBain, Director, National Chemical Laboratory, January 16, 1951, RG 6.7 S III, Box 143, F1028.

47 Work to Morison, November 4, 1955, RG 6.7, S III, Box 143, F 1030.

48 Summary of Discussion on IHD Virus Program, January 25, 1951, RG 1.1, S 464, Box 1, F 9.

49 Watson to Pandit, February 22, 1951, RG 6.7, S III, Box 143, F 1028.

50 H. H. Smith Diary Note, Friday, February 9, 1951, RG 1.1, S 464 Box 1, F 9.

51 Watson to Smith, February 22, 1951, RG 1.1, S 464, Box 1, F 9.

52 Smith to Kaur, April 25, 1951, RG 6.7, S III, Box 143, F 1028.

53 Smith to Lakshmanan, May 11, 1951, RG 1.1, S464 Box 1 F9/ RG 6.7, S III, Box 143, F 1028.

54 Watson to Pandit, April 5, 1951, RG 6.7, S III, Box 143, F 1028.

55 Warren to Lakshmanan, June 8, 1951, RG 6.7, S III, Box 143, F 1028.

56 Pandit, *My World*, 246.

57 Resolution 63101, Board of Trustees, RF, December 3–4, 1963, RG 1.2 S464 Box 95, F 900.

58 Pandit, *My World*, 245.

59 Warren to Lakshmanan, June 8, 1951, RG 6.7, S III, Box 143, F1028.

60 RF Board of Trustees Resolution, December 6 7, 1960, RG 1.2, S 464, Box 95, F 900.

61 Warren to Lakshmanan, June 8, 1951, RG 6.7, S III, Box 143, F 1028.

62 Pandit, *My World*, 245.

63 Pandit, *My World*, 246–247.

64 Pandit to Watson, January 11, 1952, RG 1.1, S 464, Box 2, F 12.

65 Kerr to Morison, January 15, 1952, RG 6.7, S III, Box 143, F 1029.

66 Kerr to Watson, December 28, 1951, RG 6.7, S III, Box 143, F 1029.

67 Warren to Lakshmanan, June 8, 1951, RG 6.7, S III, Box 143, F 1028.

68 J. A. Kerr Diary, April 21, 1955, RG 12.1 Vol. 1951–1956, Box 32.

69 Summary Report on VRC, 1955, RG 6.7, S III, Box 145, F 1055.

70 Resolution 57083, Board of Trustees, RF, April 3, 1957, RG 1.2, S 464, Box 95, F 900.

71 Resolutions of the Board of Trustees, RF, 1951–1964, RG 1.2, S 464, Box 95, F 900.

72 Kerr to B. K. Das, September 22, 1952, RG 6.7, S III, Box 144, F 1045.

73 Kerr to Krishnan, July 2, 1952, RG 6.7, S III, Box 144, F 1046.

74 Watson to Pandit, April 5, 1951, RG 6.7, S III Box 143, F 1028.

75 Smith, Inter–Office Correspondence, Proposed Virus Laboratory at Poona, India, September 11, 1951, RG 1.1, S 464, India, Box 1, F 10.

76 Summary of Discussion on IHD Virus Program, January 25, 1951, RG 1.1, S 464, Box 1, F 9.
77 Smithburn to Smith, Inter-Office Correspondence, May 23, 1951, RG 1.1, S 464, Box 1, F 9.
78 Smith to Raja, August 31, 1951, RG 1.1, S 464, Box 1, F 10.
79 Smith to Kerr, February 18, 1954, RG 1.1, S 464, Box 2, F 17.
80 Smith to Kerr, February 18, 1954, RG 1.1, S 464, Box 2, F 17.
81 Resolution 57194, Board of Trustees, RF, December 3–4, 1957; RG 1.2, S 464, Box 95, F 900.
82 Summary Report on VRC, RG 6.7, S III, Box 145, F 1055; Resolution 57194, Board of Trustees, RF, December 3–4, 1957, RG 1.2, S 464, Box 95, F 900.
83 Resolution 59189, Board of Trustees, RF, 1–2 December 1959, RG 1.2, S464, Box 95, F 900.
84 Ibid.
85 Resolution, Board of Trustees, RF, December 6–7, 1960, RG 1.2, S 464, Box 95, F 900.
86 Rockefeller Foundation Annual Report (New York, Rockefeller Foundation, 1961): 204.
87 Rockefeller Foundation Annual Report (New York, Rockefeller Foundation, 1962): 139–141.
88 Resolution 64106, Board of Trustees, RF, November 30–December 1, 1964, RG 1.2, S 464, Box 95, F 900.
89 Balfour Diary Note Wed. July 17, 1957, RG 1.2, S 464, Box 33, F 265.
90 Work to Morison August 26, 1957, RG 6.7, S III, Box 143, F 1031.
91 Balfour Diary Note Wed. July 17, 1957, RG 1.2, S 464, Box 33, F 265.
92 Resolution 57194, Board of Trustees, RF December 3–4, 1957, RG 1.2, S 464, Box 95, F 900.
93 Balfour Diary Note Wed July 17, 1957, RG 1.2, S 464, Box 33, F 265.
94 A. V. Venkasubban, Deputy Secretary, Ministry of Health, to L.R. Allen, April 30, 1958, RG 1.2, S 464, Box 94, F 894.
95 Work to Venkatsubban, May 7, 1958, RG 1.2, S 464, Box 94, F 894.
96 Resolution 57194, Board of Trustees, RF, December 3–4, 1957, RG 1.2, S 464, Box 95, F 900.
97 Resolution 58206, Board of Trustees, RF, December 2–3, 1958, RG 1.2, S 464, Box 95, F 900.
98 Resolution 59189, Board of Trustees, RF, December 1–2, 1959, RG 1.2, S 464, Box 95, F 900.
99 C. R. Anderson to Morison, January 22, 1960, RG 1.2, S464, Box 94, F 895.
100 Anderson to Morison, January 22, 1960, RG 1.2, S 464, Box 94, F 895.
101 Anderson to Morison September 13, 1960, RG 1.2, S 464, Box 94, F 895.
102 Morison to Anderson, September 20, 1960, RG 1.2, S 464, Box 94, F895.
103 Anderson to Morison, September 27, 1960, RG 1.2, S 464, Box 94, F 895.
104 Anderson to Morison, October 11, 1960, RG 1.2, S 464, Box 94, F 895.
105 Work to Dean Rusk, May 28, 1958, RG 1.2, S 464, Box 94, F 894.
106 Ibid.
107 Ibid.
108 Ibid.
109 Ibid.
110 Trapido to Morison, May 2, 1960, RG 1.1, S 464, Box 14, F 107.
111 Ibid.
112 Work to Rusk, May 28, 1958.
113 Salim Ali, *The Fall of a Sparrow* (Delhi, Oxford University Press, 1991), 144–147.

114 Trapido to Morison, February 27, 1960, RG 1.1, S 464, Box 14, F 107.
115 Trapido to Saenz, February 27, 1960, RG 1.1, S 464, Box 14, F 107.
116 Saenz to Trapido, March 7, 1960, RG 1.1, S 464, Box 14, F 107.
117 Saenz to Ali, May 13, 1959, RG 1.1, S 464, Box 14, F 106.
118 Ali to Trapido, June 4, 1959, RG 1.1 S 464 Box 14 F 106.
119 Trapido to Morison June 5, 1959, RG 1.1, S 464, Box 14, F 106.
120 Morison to Trapido, June 26, 1959, RG 1.1 S 464, Box 14, F 106.
121 Ali, *The Fall of a Sparrow*, 144–147.
122 Morison to Trapido, April 26,1960, RG 1.1, S 464, Box 14, F 107.
123 Ali, *The Fall of a Sparrow*, 144–147.
124 Nithyanand Rao, "The Seven-Decade Transnational Hunt for the Origins of a Strange Indian Disease," November 19, 2016, http://thewire.in/81210/kyasanur-kfd-rajagopalan-boshell/.
125 Lower house of the Parliament; Ali, *The Fall of a Sparrow*, 146.
126 Michael Lewis, "Scientists or Spies? Ecology in a Climate of Cold War Suspicion," *Economic and Political Weekly*, 37 (2002): 2323–2324.
127 Ibid., 2324.
128 Ibid.
129 W. Oliver Diary, Thur. November 4, 1954, RG 1.2, S 464, Box 30, F 236.
130 Administrative Correspondence, Estates and Organisations 1953, RG 6.7 Subgroup 2 MMS Programme S VRC, Poona, Box 143, F 1029.
131 Ibid.
132 Kerr, July 18, 1953, RG 12.1, Officer Diaries Vol. 1951–1956, Box 32.
133 Ibid.
134 Kerr to Smith, August 7, 1953, RG 6.7, S III, Box 144, F 1048.
135 Kerr, April 12, 1954, RG 12.1, Officer Diaries Vol. 1951–1956, Box 32.
136 These were seen confidentially by M. C. Balfour, director for the Far Eastern Region, DMPH and based in India while Pandit was handling the matter. It was the secretary to the Ministry of Health who informed Balfour that the questions were being disallowed. M.C. Balfour to A. J. Warren, May 12, 1954, RG 1.1, S 464, Box 2, F 17.
137 Balfour to Warren, May 12, 1954, RG 1.1, S 464, Box 2, F 17.
138 *New Age Weekly*, Vol. II No 30, Sunday, April 24, 1955, RG 1.1, S 464, Box 2, F 17.
139 Ibid.
140 Work to the Surgeon General with the Government of Bombay, November 7, 1955, RG 1.1, S 464, Box 3, F 22.
141 RF Board of Trustees Resolution December 3–4, 1963, RG 1.2, S 464, Box 95, F 900.
142 Anne-Emanuelle Birn and Theodore M. Brown, eds., *Comrades in Health: U.S Health Internationalists, Abroad and at Home* (New Brunswick, NJ: Rutgers University Press, 2013).
143 Ibid.
144 Tatsuo Saki and Yuh Morimoto, "The History of Infectious Diseases and Medicine," *Pathogens* 11 (October 2022): 1147, https://doi.org/10.3390/pathogens11101147.

6 Indonesian Health Policy Between the Old and the New Orders, 1949–1998

Vivek Neelakantan

Introduction

On August 17, 1955—commemorating the tenth anniversary of Indonesia's proclamation of independence—the then minister of health Johannes Leimena asserted:[1]

> With the Declaration of Independence on August 17, 1945, the formation of a government with its machine of power (police and army), its territories and population, the Republic of Indonesia came into being. The Red-White Flag was hoisted and the National Anthem was heard in the smallest and remotest places of Indonesia. It was previously gauged that this country was going to face various difficulties if it had to retain its independence. These difficulties were felt in all fields of work, including Public Health, specially before the transfer of sovereignty on December 27, 1949. Yet it may be said that Indonesians during its stage of independence showed a strong will and spirit of unity to maintain its freedom amidst hardships and difficulties and no less did it show its courage to surmount the barriers during the transition period, also in the field of health.[1]

The preceding speech illustrates the niche occupied by public health in national reconstruction in post–World War II Indonesia. Furthermore, Leimena's speech indicated continued faith placed by Indonesian leaders on the revolutionary ideology in surmounting barriers in all fields including public health.

In 1949, subsequent to the transfer of political sovereignty to the Indonesian republic, the country inherited a health system that was devastated by three-and-a-half years of War in the Pacific (1942–45) and four years of revolutionary struggle against the Dutch colonial rule. After the transfer of sovereignty—apart from the loss of Indonesian physicians due to war and revolution—Dutch doctors working in Indonesia were repatriated to the Netherlands due to the deteriorating relations between Indonesia and the Netherlands. Consequently, by 1950, Indonesia had an adverse ratio of

DOI: 10.4324/9781003318163-7

doctors, estimated at one doctor to 60,000 population (1,200 doctors for a population of 72 million).[2] To compound the situation, the country's three medical faculties at Jakarta, Surabaya and Yogyakarta graduated a modest number of 50 physicians per annum, inadequate to cope with Indonesia's population growth, estimated at 1.7 to 2 percent per annum during the 1950s.[3]

Since 2002, the evolution of healthcare in postcolonial Indonesia has received some anthropological and historical attention. Yet, a major challenge faced by historians is the compartmentalization of Indonesian history into distinct eras (*zamans*). Medical historians specializing in the Soekarno era or the *Orde Lama* (the Old Order, 1949–67) concentrate on the decolonization of healthcare, the appropriation of biomedicine by nationalist physicians, or the ways in which health became a component of post–World War II national reconstruction.[4] In contrast, scholars specializing on the Soeharto Era or the *Orde Baru* (The New Order, 1966–98) argue that despite Indonesia's noteworthy economic progress between the 1970s and the 1990s, the health of the population remained poor by regional (Southeast Asian) standards.[5] As a result of the compartmentalization of Indonesian history into *zamans*, the ways in which international developments such as the Cold War influenced the trajectory of primary healthcare remain cursorily less explored.[6]

In this chapter, I argue that the overarching theme of health policy across the Old and New Orders was national development (*pembangunan*). Whereas during the Soekarno era, *pembangunan* stood for multiple possibilities such as developments in agriculture, industry and health, during the Soeharto era, *pembangunan* was associated with state-sponsored economic development. During the 1950s, Indonesian physicians appropriated military metaphors drawn from the country's struggle against colonialism. They metaphorically referred to the campaign against disease as battles that would lead to further victories against poverty, illiteracy and disease. The mobilization of Indonesians around disease eradication involved raising the population's living standards and presenting an image of the New Indonesian as free of disease.[7] During the Soekarno era, Indonesia sought to achieve a delicate equilibrium between maintaining the country's sovereignty in health and increased openness to international aid. In contrast, during the Soeharto era, Indonesia welcomed aid from the U.S. and other international agencies in health such as the United Nations Population Fund (UNFPA) and the World Health Organization (WHO)—particularly in the field of family planning and disease eradication, respectively. The New Order administration was fixated on the regulation of family size as the means to achieve economic growth.

Health Policy in Soekarno-Era Indonesia: A Delicate Balance Between National Interests and International Health

When Indonesia attained *de jure* independence in 1949, the nascent republic faced a range of serious political problems. The Darul Islam group—that proclaimed the Islamic State of West Java in August 1949—had turned into a rebellion that affected Aceh, South Sulawesi and South Kalimantan. The fear that Javanese dominion would replace Dutch colonialism led to rebellions in West Sumatra, South Sulawesi and South Maluku into the latter part of the 1950s. Successive governments of the 1950s were faced with the challenge of raising peoples' living standards. Soon after taking office as Prime Minister in September 1950, Mohammed Natsir contended that political independence would not be automatically followed by increased prosperity.[8] Although the Natsir administration succeeded in establishing a planned framework for economic growth, it failed to secure political support. Successive governments between 1950 and 1957 were in office for too short a period to implement economic policies. During the 1950s, Indonesia made significant gains in human development due to a decline in crude death rates from 28 per 1000 in the 1930s to 26 per 1000 by the late 1950s.[9] But the decline in death rates—coupled with a jump in the annual birth rate—pushed population growth rates to 2 percent per annum by the late 1950s.

Between December 1949 and September 1950, the central government had to achieve coordination between health ministries of the seven states that constituted the United States of Indonesia, which later became the Republic of Indonesia Ministry of Health. To remedy the acute shortage of physicians, the Ministry of Health under the leadership of Leimena launched an Eleven-Point Emergency Program that consisted of (1) the control of infectious diseases (smallpox, dysentery, typhoid, cholera and plague) and endemic diseases (yaws, tuberculosis [TB], venereal diseases, trachoma and leprosy), (2) public health education, (3) expansion of curative care, (4) training of health personnel, (5) increase the supply of drugs, (6) continuation of medical research, (7) expansion of maternal and child health activities, (8) promotion of social hygiene, (9) introduction of rural health services, (10) promotion of nutrition, and (11) collaboration with international aid agencies such as the World Health Organization (WHO) and the UNICEF.[10]

The WHO, which was founded in 1948, had to come to terms with the political realities of the Cold War. A year after its foundation, the USSR and its allies (particularly Hungary, Poland, Czechoslovakia, Bulgaria, Romania and Albania) sent notifications of withdrawal from the WHO.[11] The Soviets and their allies accused the U.S. of withholding medical supplies from Eastern Europe, although these nations had paid a high price during World War II. The Soviets and their East European allies boycotted the WHO between 1949 and 1956, believing for good reason that the WHO was captive of American interests. Underlining the Soviet and its East European allies' boycott of the WHO were two diametrically opposing views of public health: between that of capitalism and that of communism. The Soviets and their allies accused the US of not recognizing the inseparable connections between social, economic and health problems.[12] In 1950, US Assistant Secretary of State for Economic Affairs Willard Thorp asserted before the American Public Health Association that a clear link existed between poverty and communism. He contended that disease and poverty must be fought because they threatened the very survival of American democracy.[13]

Between 1948 and 1952, the WHO became partially captive to U.S. national interests. It abandoned its initial vision of a collaborative community of nations and incorporated compromises over decolonization.[14] The development of WHO Regional Offices in Southeast Asia, Europe, the Eastern Mediterranean, the Western Pacific and Africa was a conspicuous feature in the organization's evolution. European powers, particularly Portugal, initially opposed regionalization in 1948 and wanted their colonies in Asia—particularly Portuguese Goa—to be made Associate Members of the newly formed WHO. In contrast, the U.S. and Latin American nations wanted the Pan American Sanitary Bureau (PASB, founded in 1902) to function as a quasi-autonomous organization. This stance provided the impetus for regionalization to prevail across the WHO. Each regional office was meant, at least in principle, to aggregate countries based on geographical proximity and similar epidemiological profile. The regional offices—quasi-independent from the WHO headquarters in Geneva—were responsible for hiring staff and interpreting WHO policies formulated at the headquarters to suit the specific requirements of the region.

The WHO Regional Office for Southeast Asia, or SEARO—the first of the WHO regional offices—was established in New Delhi with support from Indian Premier Jawaharlal Nehru in 1948. At the time, during the Second Dutch Military Action against the Indonesian republic, the Netherlands Indies Department of Health (Departemen van Gezondheid) had expressed a reservation that the birth of the SEARO would be of little benefit to Indonesia as Batavia (now known as Jakarta) was geographically closer to the would-be headquarters of the WHO Regional Office for the Western Pacific (WPRO), Manila, than New Delhi.[15] But during the Third World Health Assembly in Geneva (1950), the United States of Indonesia had decided to shift the country's membership from the WPRO to the SEARO.[16] The move was seen by Leimena as strengthening Indonesia's cooperation in international health with India, as both countries shared a common antagonism toward imperialism.[17]

Leimena was the architect of Indonesia's health policy of the 1950s. He was consecutively Minister of Health in the Cabinets of Prime Ministers Amir Sjarifuddin (July 1947–November 1949), Mohammad Hatta (January 1948–July 1949), Natsir (September 1950-March 1951), Soekiman (April 1951–April 1952), Wilopo (April 1952–July 1953) and Burnahuddin Harahap (August 1955–March 1956), except for the brief period between 1953 and 1955 when Lie Kiat Teng served in this position. Leimena's outlook on public health—while closely aligned to the prescriptions of the WHO—sought to maximize international funding for the Ministry of Health's pilot health projects—while cautiously balancing Indonesia's hard-won political sovereignty and nationalist rhetoric that stressed on economic self-sufficiency ("berdiri di atas kaki sendiri").

Leimena's political philosophy—an eclectic blend of Christianity, nationalist ideology and internationalism—influenced his outlook on health. As an Ambonese Christian, he embodied the ideal of unity in diversity ("bhinneka tunggal eka") of the Indonesian archipelago. Appropriating biblical metaphors, he illustrated health challenges faced by the international community during the Cold War:

> The aftermath of two world wars, the tensions incident to the present cold war, and the threat of atomic world disaster, have produced a profound popular yearning for peace. This desire is not limited to the great powers. It is especially characteristic of the newly independent nations. Starting late in the technological race, these young nations recognise that only if there is an extended period of world peace can they develop their internal economies so as to supply their peoples with an abundant living. They must raise the national standards of living by improving social and economic conditions. They must provide relief from hunger, poverty and preventable disease. Thus these young national Davids are pitting themselves against four Goliaths: Ignorance, Poverty, Disease, and Unemployment. Their slender slingshot is effective thought and planning; the stone with which they must slay the enemy is hard work.[18]

Furthermore, Leimena was of the conviction that as poverty and illiteracy were the breeding grounds of Communist ideology, Indonesia needed to undertake rural development projects calculated to raise peoples' living standards.[19]

Leimena's thinking on public health resonated with that of American bacteriologist Charles-Edward Amory Winslow, who was a consultant to the WHO in the 1950s and published the treatise *Cost of Sickness and the Price of Health*.[20] In the treatise, Winslow highlighted a correlation between poverty and disease. Elaborating on Winslow's correlation between poverty and disease, Leimena contended that disease and poverty constituted a vicious circle. A sick person became poor, and poverty accounted for the disease becoming worse, which, in turn, entailed greater poverty. Health activities without amelioration of socioeconomic conditions of the people could create an unbalanced situation in the community.[21] Leimena's thinking on public health materialized in his somewhat ambitious Bandung Plan—that was initially implemented as a pilot health project in the regency of Bandung in 1951—and later extended throughout Indonesia by 1954.

The Bandung Plan was based on the principle of integrating curative and preventive care. The plan emphasized strengthening the health services in rural areas. The plan established a referral system for curative care, focused on the village (*desa*) and subdistrict (*kecamatan*). It conceptualized healthcare delivery at four levels: (a) the setting up of one health center per subdistrict, (b) the establishment of one new healthcare center every two years, (c) the building of auxiliary hospitals in the district headquarters, and (d) the establishment of auxiliary hospitals in all district headquarters within five years.[22] The implementation of the Bandung Plan was decentralized to the provinces and regencies although the Ministry of Health dictated the health policies.[23] The plan devolved the administration of preventive hygiene work to the villages. The hygiene assistant (*djuru hygiene*) would work in close collaboration with the village officials in the implementation of public health education and the sanitation of houses and markets. At the village level, Leimena intended to mobilize the population on the basis of mutual cooperation (*gotong rojong*) to establish a *desa* hygiene service. But the ability of local governments to carry out health programs delegated by the central government was contingent on their budgets. Financing the Bandung Plan was a thorny issue between the central and local governments as not all regencies were able to support the integration of preventive and curative health activities.[24]

After being successfully implemented in the regency of Bandung, the Plan halved the prevalence of infant mortality in the city between 1951 and 1956.[25] In contrast, the infant mortality figures for the Bandung regency during the same period remained unchanged due to acute shortage of doctors in rural areas of the regency. In 1951—supported by the Soekiman cabinet—the Indonesian House of Representatives (Dewan Perwakilan Rakjat or DPR) enacted three controversial laws to regulate licensing of physicians and dentists, equitable distribution of physicians across the archipelago and private practice.[26] The laws stipulated that those physicians desirous of establishing private practice had to work in the public service for three years before they would be granted a license (*surat idzin*). Newly graduated doctors and nurses could not practice in areas having surplus medical personnel, as determined by the Indonesian Ministry of Health, and therefore were disallowed from private practice.[27] The proposals to enact the three laws were met with stiff resistance from medical students at Universitas Indonesia as the burden for ensuring the equitable distribution of physicians fell squarely on newly graduated physicians. But legislative measures in themselves failed to redress the poor graduation rates from the country's medical schools at Jakarta, Surabaya and Yogyakarta.

To remedy the shortfall of physicians, the Bandung Plan enlisted the assistance of missionary hospitals that were placed under the supervision of the regency government for the provision of curative healthcare. The Wilopo cabinet had introduced a controversial legislation, under the direction of Leimena—Indonesian Law No. 18, 1953—which stated that the state would be responsible for the attainment for the highest possible level of health for the Indonesian people by subsidizing the construction of private hospitals that catered to the needs of the poor who could not otherwise access curative care.[28] In Makele, on the island of Sulawesi, Christian missionary polyclinics that served only a few patients were subsidized despite the fact that Makele lacked a qualified doctor.[29] Locals from South Sulawesi—a province with a Muslim majority—were hesitant to use missionary hospitals on religious grounds and, instead, turned to folk healers (*tabibs*) who offered free treatment.[30] The DPR discussions indicated dissensus—particularly between the Islamist Masjumi and Parkindo (Indonesian Christian Party)—members of the ruling Indonesian National Party (PNI) coalition, on one hand, and the Indonesian Communist Party (PKI) on the other, regarding subsidizing the treatment of the poor in missionary hospitals.

The participation of provincial governments in the implementation of the Bandung Plan was perfunctory. Although the government offered subsidies to private, especially missionary hospitals, provincial governments were not enlisted in the management of these institutions.[31] A major impediment that frustrated the Bandung Plan's objectives of integrating preventive and curative health measures was the poor remuneration of physicians, nurses and para-medical personnel who worked in rural areas, particularly in the outer islands of Sumatra, Kalimantan and Sulawesi. In Sumatra, many Dutch physicians serving the plantations had departed for the Netherlands during the Dutch Military Action (1947–48).[32] In the residency of Bengkulu, with an estimated population of 300,000, two physicians served an area of roughly 500 square kilometers.[33] The Bandung Plan devolved the payment of salaries of health personnel to the local governments. In the province of South Sulawesi, for example, smallpox vaccinators received a pittance of 0.50 rupiahs.[34]

The preventive component of the Bandung Plan chiefly consisted of the control of endemic diseases such as malaria—that Leimena symbolically referred to as "enemy number one" (*musuh nomor pertama*) of the Indonesian people.[35] Between 1949 and 1965, malaria eradication in Indonesia was presented within the framework of President Soekarno's *pembangunan* ideology. President Soekarno conceptualized *pembangunan* to articulate Indonesia's aspirations for a brighter future after three-and-a-half centuries of Dutch colonialism.[36] Soekarno's notion of *pembangunan* was holistic and embraced advancements in public health, communications, the construction of monuments, the development of a strong military and a favorable balance of trade for Indonesia, indicating to the world that the country was capable of standing on its own two feet (*berdiri di atas kaki sendiri*).[37] For Soekarno, the meaning of freedom (*merdeka*) was reflected in the Javanese aphorism "subur, kang sarwa tinandur, murah, kang sarwa tinuku" (prosperity in which everyone was assured of their basic needs).[38]

The disease etiologies constructed by Indonesian physicians sought to correlate the prevalence of disease with debilitation of the nation's workforce leading to lowered agricultural productivity and starvation. Within the framework of *pembangunan* malaria was cast as a ghost or *hantu* that haunted the coastal areas of the archipelago and its hinterland, causing malnutrition among children.[39]

Regarding the common denominator underlying malaria control efforts of the Indonesian government, the WHO and the U.S. were of the conviction that malaria control would lead to enhanced economic productivity. During the 1950s, the U.S. wrestled with the USSR and China for global dominance and influence in newly independent nations of Asia and Africa to win the hearts and minds of the local population.[40] Technical assistance programs to emerging nations became weapons in the battle against communist ideology. These programs were seen as ways to break the causal link between poverty and disease on which communist ideology thrived. In his 1955 speech, U.S. president Dwight Eisenhower inaugurated the Global Malaria Eradication Campaign:

> Of all diseases, malaria, which attacked 200 million people and killed two million, is probably the worst source of poverty and misery. We are undertaking, in cooperation with the World Health Organization and countries affected, a five-year plan to abolish malaria once for all from the face of the earth.[41]

In his speech, Eisenhower observed that improved health cut down poverty and misery, supposedly well-known breeding grounds of disorder and communism. The speech attested to the ways in which malaria eradication became enmeshed in the U.S. Cold War propaganda.

During the early 1950s, Indonesia implemented malaria control measures through a combination of insecticide spraying, mass quininization of affected populations and draining of swamps. But these measures were unworkable due to the high capital expenditure involved.[42] But the control campaigns began to eventually rely on the insecticide DDT by the mid-1950s. Although the malaria control program was centralized under the control of the Malaria Control Institute in Jakarta, provincial health inspectors had actual control over the implementation of anti-malarial activities in territories under their jurisdiction. But they were constrained by dependence upon Jakarta for timely disbursement of funds.[43]

By 1958, Indonesia implemented its national malaria eradication program with assistance from the U.S. and the WHO. It was highly successful until 1963 when mosquitoes developed resistance to DDT. Organizational challenges included compliance with local administrative procedures for replacing spare parts of DDT sprayers or worn tires of vehicles that delayed the progress of the campaign. In 1959, subsequent to Soekarno's suspension of parliamentary institutions, the Manifesto Politik doctrine—including satisfaction of the basic needs of the people and struggle against imperialism—was introduced to further the cause of Indonesian socialism.[44] Consequently, U.S. funding for Indonesia's malaria eradication program halved from $10 million (1958–59) to $5 million (1959–60).[45] The International Cooperation Administration (ICA, operating from 1955–61)—responsible for US foreign assistance—made an appeal to Prime Minister Djuanda Kartawidjaja to slow down the program whereas the Minister of Health Satrio was fighting to expand it.[46] The SEARO Regional Director C. Mani had to balance between ensuring Indonesian compliance with ICA directives that granted greater autonomy to the National Malaria Eradication Program and Satrio's vision of expanding coverage of the malaria eradication program.[47]

The overall policy of the U.S. toward Indonesia (between 1955 and 1965) was to maintain and strengthen economic stability and prevent Indonesia's entry into the Soviet orbit. In the aftermath of the Asian African Conference at Bandung (1955) that gave rise to the proverbial Non-Aligned Movement (1964), the USSR became particularly interested in providing political support to Indonesia. The Soviet–Indonesian relationship was influenced by President Soekarno's Marhaenist ideology that emphasized socio-nationalism, social democracy, *gotong rojong* and socialism.[48] Although Indonesia was not a strictly socialist state, its condemnation of colonialism drew attention from the USSR at the Bandung Conference.[49] In the aftermath of Bandung, the USSR extended an unconditional aid of US$250 million for the Indonesian Five-Year-Plan.[50]

By 1960, the Soviets used health as a tool of political propaganda. D.D. Venediktov, the then Soviet deputy health minister contended that the problem of health in newly developed nations of Asia and Africa was essentially a political question. To this effect, Soviets aided preventive health campaigns such as mass vaccinations against smallpox and cholera across Asia and Africa.[51] In the Indonesian context, the USSR sponsored the official visit of Satrio to Moscow to study the Soviet health system.[52] Despite considerable Soviet investment in Indonesia, totaling to 789 million rubles (1959–65), the Indonesians completed only one health project: the Soviet-Indonesian Hospital of Friendship (Rumah Sakit Persahabatan).[53] Substantial communist gains in the first Indonesian election (1955), nonetheless, had disrupted U.S. strategic interests in the country.[54]

At the time, Soekarno was preoccupied with restoring national unity even at the expense of Communist participation in the government. He used Guided Democracy (Demokrasi Terpimpin) to further his political ends, given the context of political instability in the wake of the Sumatra–Sulawesi insurrections (1957)—a move that eventually led to the failure of constitutional democracy in Indonesia.[55] The U.S. had calculated that an abrupt termination of technical assistance would strengthen the communists on Java.[56] During the late 1950s, American aid in Indonesia was mostly focused on the Outer Islands, particularly Sumatra. At the time, the U.S. collaborated with Australia in an aborted attempt to establish a medical school at Bukittinggi in Western Sumatra during the West Sumatran Rebellion (1956–60) led by the moderate Islamist Masjumi Party.[57]

Foreign aid was a sensitive issue in Indonesian politics during the Soekarno Era. During his address to the U.S. Congress in 1956, Soekarno appreciated U.S. offers of technical assistance for Indonesia: "We will accept aid with the great appreciation that may come to us, from whatever quarter it may come for that assistance will lighten our burdens and shorten our struggles. Such assistance is not one-sided but is of mutual benefit."[58] The quote highlights underlying reservations within Indonesia that an uncritical acceptance of foreign aid would lead to an erosion of the country's hard-earned political sovereignty. During the 1950s, Soekarno faced several political challenges such as an uneasy coalescence between the army, the Islamist parties and the PKI and resolving national problems such as poverty and food security. The causal linkages between overpopulation, resource exhaustion, hunger and political instability were not yet apparent to Soekarno during the early 1950s.

Discussions pertaining to family planning during the Soekarno era could be reduced to two propositions: first, poverty and high fertility continued to kill mothers, and second, poverty could be overcome through economic planning.[59] Julie Sulianti Saroso (1917–91)—technical director of maternal and child health during the early 1950s—advocated the use of family planning to prevent maternal mortality.[60] Funded by a WHO Fellowship to study the functioning of maternal and child health policies of Sweden, Saroso observed that family planning programs were implemented through the country's district health centers. In a Radio Republik Indonesia broadcast, Saroso was open about the use of birth control as a means to prevent maternal mortality. But Vice President Mohammad Hatta was outraged by Saroso's open advocacy for using birth control to limit family size as, according to him, it offended the cultural and religious sensibilities of the Indonesian population.[61]

Soekarno therefore adopted a nuanced stance relating to the use of birth control to limit family size.[62] He admitted that Indonesia's population was growing at the rate of one million per annum, increasing the pressure of population on land. The President saw Indonesia's growing population as the key to harnessing the country's natural resources. Soekarno approached the population problem with a vision to transform Indonesia from a plantation-based economy based on subsistence agriculture to a self-supporting socialist economy that was capable of standing on its own feet ("berdiri di atas kaki sendiri") based on industrialization.[63] Based on Soekarno's claim during the mid-1950s that Indonesia was capable of feeding a population of 250 million, foreign journalists such as Louis Fischer portrayed the President as "pro-natalist."[64] Although Soekarno was privately supportive of birth control to protect maternal health, as President of Indonesia, he did not want to be seen as accepting advice from foreigners on family planning programs that were perceived at the time to be associated with immorality.[65] Family planning during the Soekarno era consisted of isolated demonstration projects such as the Cerme Project—first implemented in the subdistrict of Cerme in East Java in 1961—supported by the Population Council and the local governments whereas the involvement of the central government was minimal.[66] In contrast, family planning became the cornerstone of state policy during the New Order by 1968.

What distinguished public health and planning in the Soekarno era from the succeeding Soeharto era was the urgency and sense of revolution.[67] Soekarno's socialist politics and internationalism—reflected in the Final Communiqué of the Bandung Conference—exhorted newly independent Asian and African countries to build a new world order based on self-determination, human rights, solidarity and peace.[68] Soekarno played a symbolic role in forging an anti-imperialist front that consisted of progressive states and popu-lar movements. He coined the term "New Emerging Forces" to describe the new political formations, governments and movements, which wanted to build a new global order, as opposed to the "Old Established Forces," or OLDEFOS, whose constituents were not only the former colonial powers but also the United States and the conservative elite in postcolonial societies.[69] The Second Afro-Asian Congress of Pediatrics convened in Jakarta in 1964 reflected Soekarno's idea of New Emerging Forces that the cooperation of Asian and African nations was not only political but also in all fields of endeavor, including health.[70]

In 1964, Soekarno bluntly told the U.S. Ambassador to Indonesia Howard Jones, "To Hell with Your Aid."[71] The statement was issued in the wake of Indonesia's confrontation with Malaysia (1961–66) that ended only with the overthrow of the Old Order. At the time, the U.S. attached the condition to its aid that Indonesia end its confrontation with Malaysia. Soekarno responded by withdrawing Indonesia from the United Nations and its specialized agen-cies, including the World Bank, the FAO (Food and Agricultural Organiza-tion), the WHO and UNICEF. The decision jeopardized international assistance earmarked for Indonesia by these specialized agencies estimated at US$50 million.[72]

Between 1959 and 1965, Soekarno's unrealistic economic policies such as enforcing unreachable production targets, compulsory rice sales and infla-tion estimated at 200 percent per annum increased the privations of the people.[73] In Javanese and Balinese villages such as Ktut Kantor, villagers remembered the end of the Soekarno era as an "era of poverty."[74] In central Java, hunger edema rates had increased such that local officials estimated at least 30,000 individuals in the area of Gunung Kidul alone in 1963 were undernourished.[75]

The central government launched the Operation to Eradicate Ignorance in Nutrition in 1964, based on mass mobilization of the masses invoking the slogan "strong nation is a healthy nation" (rakjat sehat, negara kuat), during the military confrontation with Malaysia. Although the campaign was success-ful in mobilizing women's organizations such as the Indonesian Women's Congress (Kongres Wanita Indonesia), the operation failed in its mission to introduce diversity in peoples' diets due to hyperinflation.[76] Incidentally, Soekarno's inability to redress food insecurity in Indonesia led to his downfall in 1965.

Between 1957 and 1965, Soekarno's authoritarian tendencies, supported partly by the military and vested interests within the ruling class, pushed Indonesia beyond the limits of its economic base, social structure and polit-ical institutions. In the name of continuing the revolution, Soekarno nation-alized foreign enterprises in Indonesia and increased the power of the military. Then, as a counterweight to the military, he supported the PKI. The "crash-through or crash" approach led to the greatest disaster in the nation's history.[77]

Healthcare in the Soeharto Era: The Illusion of Development

Late on the evening of September 30, 1965, army units led by Col. General Untung launched a limited coup in Jakarta. The coup intended to remove a council of generals alleged to be plotting to remove Soekarno with the help of the U.S. and Britain. The dramatic murder of six military generals, allegedly by the PKI gave General Soeharto the opportunity to move to the center of Indonesian political life.[78] Conservative forces and public opinion in Indonesia attributed the coup to PKI, and the Soeharto government generally enforced that view.[79] Evidence of direct PKI involvement in planning the coup, however, was slender and was mainly based on dubious confessions and on testimony concerning a so-called Biro Khusus (Special Bureau) of the PKI formed to recruit military officers for the party.[80] Indonesian students—who styled themselves "Angkatan 66" (generation of 1966)—demanded the extirpation of communism, the end of corruption, and lower prices for essentials.[81] Between 1966 and 1968, Soeharto consolidated his power. In 1968, he was declared president, starting the New Order. The military dominated the government for the next three decades.

U.S. support for the New Order regime was forthcoming after they were convinced of Soeharto's anti-communist credentials.[82] After Soeharto acceded to U.S. demands to open Indonesia's borders for U.S. corporations, the country received generous financial aid and generous debt rescheduling.[83] Indonesia rejoined the World Bank in 1967. On July 3, 1971, Indonesia held its first elections under the New Order. Suharto's victory had inaugurated an era of accelerated modernization in which the military-technocratic alliance would depoliticize the "floating masses" down to the level of rapid export-led growth and the creation of a new national identity based on a collective commitment to economic growth.[84] For over three decades (1966–1998), the New Order regime promised stability and order in the name of development, rationalized state violence and repressed the Indonesian labor movement, civil society and students' unions.

During the New Order, Indonesian authorities interpreted *pembangunan* in the light of the country's economic and political crisis that led to the downfall of Soekarno, purged it of its nationalistic overtones and framed development as a technical and apolitical process.[85] With the PKI crushed and the weakening of other political parties, New Order military officials and technocrats adapted American modernization theory to suit their own needs so that Indonesia could try and use the resources from the modern West and synthesize it with the country's premodern social, culture and religious traditions.[86] Indonesia opened for foreign investment. President Soeharto styled himself as "father of development" (*bapak pembangunan*). The New Order era, however, was beset by contradictions. Whereas living standards of the people improved, there was a rise in corruption and random state-sanctioned violence. Under Soeharto's presidency, poverty fell from 45 percent in 1970 to 11 percent in 1996, life expectancy rose from 47 in 1966 to 67 by 1997.[87] By

1985, the FAO awarded him a gold medal for helping Indonesia achieve self-sufficiency in the production of rice.

Health policy of the New Order bore the imprint of Moluccan physician Gerrit Siwabessy, who officiated as the Minister of Health between 1966 and 1978. When he took up his official position, he removed all employees within the Ministry of Health alleged to hold sympathies toward the PKI and began the delicate task of rebuilding Indonesia's relations with the WHO, which had experienced some strain during the late 1950s.[88] In 1968, he convened a National Health Conference in which he proposed to expand healthcare across the archipelago through the provision of community health centers or *Puskesmas* at the subdistrict level (a similar proposal earlier made by Leimena in 1951).[89] His proposals were echoed in Indonesia's Repelita I (First Five-Year Development Plan under the New Order, 1969–74). During the Second Five Year Development Plan (Repelita II), with a view toward increasing the efficiency of the Department of Health (DEPKES), Siwabessy proposed the integration of preventive and curative health facilities and established a *Puskesmas* in each subdistrict toward the end of the 1970s.[90]

The establishment of *Puskesmas* in each subdistrict across Indonesia by the late 1970s was concomitant with the rise of the Primary Healthcare paradigm worldwide. In 1978, the WHO convened the Alma Ata Conference on Primary Healthcare. After the U.S. and the WHO jointly sponsored malaria eradication program failed in 1969, the Soviets proposed an alternative strategy for strengthening health services based on community participation.[91] The conference's conclusions were comparable to the findings of the League of Nations Health Organization's Intergovernmental Conference on Far-Eastern Countries on Rural Hygiene held in Bandung in1937.[92]

The Indonesian delegates to the Alma Ata Conference elaborated on primary healthcare initiatives already undertaken in their country during the 1960s and 1970s. Between 1966 and 1974, Indonesian physician Gunawan Nugroho designed an innovative health program, based on community participation. In the village of Bejagah in central Java, he observed chronic malnutrition.[93] Instead of medical treatment, Nugroho established a village development committee that introduced new high-yielding varieties of rice. Furthermore, the committee invited the government to educate farmers about using fertilizers to increase the yield. Through food-for-work programs where labor was provided in return for Bulgar wheat, the irrigation channels were improved drastically. Between 1966 and 1970, agricultural yields almost doubled and infant mortality declined.[94]

In the second case, Nugroho introduced a pilot community health insurance scheme (*dana sehat*) in Solo, Central Java, during the early 1970s.[95] Nugroho encouraged the community to assess its own health problems and potential solutions. Each villager paid only 1.5 cents (5 rupiahs) to the insurance scheme.[96] In the scheme whereas the villagers met nearly half their healthcare expenditure, the rest was contributed by the central government. Nugroho's health initiatives were among several initiatives pioneered by physicians at the grassroots level that inspired the WHO's formulation of the Primary Healthcare approach at Alma Ata in 1978.

Physician Januar Achmad—who served for ten years in a *puskesmas* in Kaliangkrik, Central Java—contended that economic growth during the New Order era did not translate into improvements in health conditions. There were some programmatic successes such as the intensification of rice cultivation, universal immunization and family planning. Between 1960 and 1993, infant mortality was cut by more than half, from 139 per 1000 births (1960) to 56 per 1000 births (1993).[97] Yet, Indonesian health indicators during the New Order hid disparities across provinces. According to the Central Bureau of Statistics (1994) estimate, Indonesian infant mortality rates varied from 40 per 1000 in Jakarta to 145 per 1000 in West Nusa Tenggara. Between 1969 and 1977, the number of *puskesmas* increased from 1058 (1969) to 4029 (1977).[98] In fact the construction of *puskesmas* exceeded the expectations of Repelita II. But the challenge was to increase staffing and utilization of health services. The under-utilization of health services could be attributed to Indonesians' preference for traditional medicine. By 1977, the New Order Regime introduced Village Community Health Development ("Pembangunan Kesehatan Masyarakat Desa") to meet the needs of the rural poor. But the program was centralized under the supervision of the Ministry of Home Affairs. Health officials, then, had little control over the program.

The most noteworthy public health success registered by the New Order administration was the eradication of smallpox. In 1958—as the USSR proposed the global eradication of smallpox at the Eleventh World Health Assembly—Indonesia had the second-highest incidence of smallpox in the world after India.[99] The prevention of smallpox at the time consisted of ad hoc mass vaccination campaigns of the population in endemic areas to increase herd immunity. But the fragmentation of public health responsibilities between the central and provincial governments, on one hand, and political uncertainties towards the end of the Soekarno era, on the other, interrupted smallpox vaccinations between 1965 and 1967. Between 1968 and 1974, Indonesia implemented eradication through a combination of mass vaccination of uninfected individuals; and, detection of infected cases (surveillance) and containment. The eradication campaign was implemented through a chain-of-command reporting style in which the upper echelons of the bureaucracy at the Directorate General of Communicable Diseases (Department of Health, Jakarta) compelled lower-level bureaucracy at the village (*desa*), subdistrict (*kecamatan*) and regency (*kabupaten*) to notify about suspected cases.[100] The centralized strategies were successful and the country managed to eradicate smallpox by 1974.

The New Order regime was concerned with bolstering economic growth, political stability and social control across Indonesia. In 1966, Ali Sadikin, the governor of Jakarta, linked urban problems to population growth. He challenged the PKBI (Indonesian Planned Parenthood Association, founded in 1957) to devise a project that would ease population growth in Jakarta.[101]

Sadikin was the first Indonesian leader to commit state resources to family planning. The Jakarta Pilot Project, the country's first family planning project was active in 1967.[102] Following the success of the Jakarta Project, Soeharto institutionalized the national family planning program in 1968. In 1970, the National Family Planning Coordinating Board (BKKBN) was established to coordinate family planning activities across government departments and non-governmental organizations. Foreign donors invested heavily in the BKKBN to build a strong bureaucracy capable of handling the logistics, family promotion and training tasks that were beyond the capabilities of the departments of Health and Information.[103]

The chief challenge encountered by the BKKBN was to overcome community resistance. Demographer Donald Warwick's interview with villagers between 1979 and 1984 indicated that eligible couples were unwilling to join the family planning program as they thought that participation in the program was shameful.[104] Muslim leaders in villages shaped the public opinion on family planning as prospective acceptors turned to them for advice with respect to the program's moral acceptability.[105] In East and West Java, for example, Muslim leaders were initially hostile when the program was first introduced in 1974. In contrast, the province of South Sulawesi, a strongly Muslim region, witnessed little opposition to the program on religious grounds.[106] The government, in turn, allayed the fears of religious leaders by omitting two methods of fertility control opposed by pious Muslims, namely, abortion and sterilization. Furthermore, wherever religious opposition to family planning was a problem, authorities would cite a non-binding legal opinion on a point of Islamic law (*fatwa*) from the Ministry of Religious Affairs to state that fertility control was a religious obligation.

A major shortcoming in Indonesia's family planning program was the acute shortage of physicians and health personnel. Even in 1977, Indonesia had an adverse physician-to-population ratio, estimated at one physician per 21,000 population.[107] But there was spectacular growth in the number of family planning clinics from 116 PKBI clinics, sprinkled across Java and Bali in 1967 to more than 2,700 clinics managed by the government in 1976.[108] One of BKKBN's controversial measures had been the target system whereby authorities sent thousands of village functionaries searching for acceptors.[109] Bureaucrats sometimes applied undue pressure on women to participate in the program. By 1977, the BKKBN propaganda shifted from "space the children" and the four-child family to "stop at two," a target promoted by Indonesia's "Zero Population Growth" movement.[110] The BKKBN's pilot projects increasingly emphasized training its fieldworkers in basic infant care and nutrition. These training initiatives demonstrated the importance of integrating family planning services within the health system. Between 1972 and 1977, total fertility rate in Java and Bali dropped from 5.8 to 3.8 children per woman.[111]

During the early and mid-1990s, Indonesian newspapers published commentaries related to the detrimental effects of progress (*kemajuan*). Lifestyle and degenerative diseases such as Type 2 diabetes became more prevalent among Indonesians.[112] Anthropologist Steve Ferzacca interprets these events as indirect expressions of dissatisfaction with the New Order regime.[113]

The demise of the New Order political structure by May 1998 could be attributed to the demise of the Cold War in 1991. Soeharto did not seem to realize that with the end of the Cold War, his position as a staunch anti-Communist ally of the U.S. had greatly diminished in value.[114] The post–Cold War emphasis on democratization, human rights, environmental protection, transparency and good governance went against the New Order regime's political and economic interests. The New Order adopted a defensive attitude toward international criticisms during the 1990s when external aid was linked to individual countries' human rights records. Soeharto also failed to understand that globalization had led to the emergence of an increasingly critical civil society in Indonesia that demanded increased accountability and transparency in governance. As the Indonesian government faced domestic and international pressures to reform, it was unable to withstand the impact of the 1997 economic crisis that swept across East and Southeast Asia. The resignation of President Soeharto on May 21, 1998, amid student riots ushered in the *Reformasi* or the Era of Reform.

Conclusion

Having analyzed the health policy of Indonesia across the Soekarno and the Soeharto Eras (1949–98), one can conclude that the Soekarno era was a period of unfulfilled aspirations despite some successes in Indonesian public health. The first five years following the transfer of power from the Dutch to the Indonesian republic could be termed a period of optimism. In 1955, the mean life expectancy of Indonesians was 50 years, approximately 10 years higher than in the 1930s. The number of physicians doubled from 800 in 1945 to 1600 in 1955.[115] By 1955, Leimena was confident that the overall state of health in Indonesia at the time could be regarded as "satisfactory."[116]

Even during the early 1950s, however, the optimism of the Ministry of Health could not be justified. Indonesian writer Pramoedya Ananta Toer depicted a picture not of development but ever-present death in his short story "My Kampung," when the campaign against endemic diseases was underway. In a sarcastic vein he wrote:

> A small guerrilla squad that is cautious is not likely to lose ten people in two years, yet in my peaceful kampung with its smell and conditions, people die one after another. They die a cheap death, friend. Like this, at the back of my house, soon after I started living in Kebun Djahe Kober, one person died because of a chronic venereal disease. After that, a woman died in the very same house after saying: "You see, I'm not afraid to die, it's better than living like this." And so she died, calm and happy

after sleeping in her platform bed for two months straight, not wanting to cook and not wanting to eat if food did not come to her.[117]

Furthermore, Toer pointed out that his disease-prone kampung (urban slum) in Jakarta was not more than 500 meters from the national palace, making the contrast between the country's political elite and the urban poor even more jarring. The preceding quote highlighted the indifference of the postcolonial state towards ameliorating peoples' socioeconomic conditions.

The Soekarno-era commitment to healthcare was enshrined in the Basic Law of Health, No. 9 (Undang Undang Nomor 9, Tentang Pokok Pokok Kesehatan), 1960 and signed by Prime Minister Djuanda Kartawidjaja. The law stated that the health of the people played an important role in the completion of the national revolution and the establishment of a socialist society.[118] Furthermore, the law guaranteed the highest possible standard of health for the Indonesian citizen. But the state commitment to guaranteeing the best possible level of health for Indonesian citizens health during the 1950s was hampered due to food insecurity, hyperinflation, military confrontation with Malaysia and challenge to the authority of the central government, particularly evident in the anti-communist West Sumatra Rebellion.

During the Soekarno era, as foreign aid was a sensitive issue in Indonesian politics, the administration tried to achieve a delicate equilibrium between maintaining the country's sovereignty in health and increased openness toward international technical assistance. In the 1950s—given the association of the family planning program with international aid agencies and opposition from Islamist parties on religious and moral grounds—Soekarno was reluctant to endorse birth control as a means of family planning. As President of Indonesia, he did not want to be seen as accepting prescriptions of American aid agencies for fear of getting entangled in Cold War politics.

Public health achievements of the Soekarno era may pale in comparison to the Soeharto era. Yet, the revolutionary rhetoric of the Soekarno era as embodied in the aphorism "a strong nation is a healthy nation" (rakjat sehat, negara kuat) and decentralized health governance have influenced health planning from 1999 to the present.

During the Soeharto era, health was not perceived as a security risk for the state. On the contrary, population explosion was considered as a threat to internal security. The New Order regime prioritized clothing (*sandang*), food (*pangan*) and shelter (*papan*) based on the Javanese conception of a peaceful and harmonious life.[119] The Ministry of Interior was used as the main pillar by the central government to implement health policies up to the village level such that the local government was accountable to the Ministry of Interior and not to the Ministry of Health. The user fees from *puskesmas* were the second-most important source of revenue for the local governments, but a big proportion of this revenue was used for non-health purposes.[120]

The New Order regime maintained the balance of power by distributing lucrative monopolies in the Indonesian economy between the military (that guaranteed the stability of his regime) and the capital-rich private enterprise (that contributed to investment and job creation). But by the early 1990s, Soeharto's family became more predatory by sucking up economic opportunities. As millions of ordinary Indonesians were lifted out of poverty, they began to demand more public services. During the early 1990s, the country's social security funds were used as slush funds to buy political opponents to Soeharto's shaky regime and fund the most basic health services.[121] In May 1998, after Soeharto abdicated as president, he was replaced by Vice President B.J. Habibie, a technocrat who tried to mitigate the worst impact of the Asian financial crisis (1997–98) by negotiating a loan from the Asian Development Bank. The loan enabled the government to issue health cards that allowed poor families to seek free healthcare.

Disease Control in Decentralized Indonesia: From H5N1 Avian Influenza to COVID-19

From 2001 onward, Indonesia embarked on administrative decentralization to relieve the pressure that was building up against decades of centralization that seemed to extract resources from the resource-rich Outer Islands for the benefit of densely populated Java. Administrative responsibilities for most state functions were devolved to districts. The devolution of administrative functions to local governments came at a time when overseas funding for centrally directed health programs ended. Although decentralization has promoted local ownership of health priorities across Indonesia and has tailored health interventions to suit local contexts, decentralization has also weakened centralized disease surveillance. Diseases such as H5N1 avian influenza and COVID-19 do not recognize political borders.

Indonesia came under fire internationally in 2007 and 2008 when the then Minister of Health Siti Fadilah Supari refused to share the country's avian influenza samples with the WHO. Whereas the international community presented the H5N1 outbreak as a humanitarian endeavor that required cooperation, Supari argued that the nation and the international community, represented by the WHO should hold rights to viral samples.[122] She expressed strong reservations with respect to international drug companies profiteering from the humanitarianism of sample-sharing countries such as Indonesia. To promote Supari's argument, Indonesia hosted a high-level meeting of the WHO and national health ministers in 2007 during which delegates discussed how avian influenza samples could be shared fairly and equitably.[123] Under Supari's global leadership, Indonesia was again projected as the leader of the postcolonial world, reviving the legacy of the Asian African Conference at Bandung (1955) that resisted imperialism and Cold War alignments.[124]

The archipelagic nature of Indonesia and decentralized health governance posed special challenges to the management of the novel coronavirus in February 2020 that in turn, led to an indecisive response to the coronavirus crisis from the center. Between January and February 2020—as the novel coronavirus ravaged China—Indonesia claimed it had zero coronavirus cases. But local newspapers such as *The Jakarta Post* claimed that 13 suspected coronavirus cases were reported from across the Indonesian archipelago.[125] Indonesia's neighbors, particularly Singapore, had confirmed coronavirus cases in early 2020. But the former Indonesian Minister of Health, Terawan Agus Putranto, a retired military physician, tried to downplay the crisis. He attributed the coronavirus-free status of Indonesia to prayers. A Harvard study, led by Marc Lipsitch, analyzed air traffic density out of Wuhan and inferred that Indonesia might have missed coronavirus cases. Putranto dismissed the study as "insulting." [126] The economy-first approach of President Joko Widodo (Jokowi) sought to capitalize on Indonesia's supposedly COVID-free status and promote the country as a tourist destination. The central government was adopting a developmentalist mindset at the expense of what was a public health emergency.[127]

Given the lackadaisical approach of the central administration to the COVID-19 crisis, provincial and local governments were pushed to implement their own versions of a lockdown. Indonesia's early responses to the pandemic were politicized. On February 25, 2020, Governor of Jakarta Anies Baswedan—a contender for the 2024 presidential elections—insisted that local governments increase vigilance against coronavirus and implemented his own version of a lockdown.[128] On March 2, 2020, Jokowi officially declared the first two COVID-19 cases in Indonesia. On March 20, 2020, Baswedan declared a state of emergency in Jakarta and implemented large-scale social restrictions or Pembatasan Sosial Berskala Besar (PSBB). Jokowi rebuked Baswedan's decree by stating that only the central government could impose PSBB, based on data submitted by provincial governments, documenting the increase in COVID-19 cases. Consequently, a hotchpotch of PSBB restrictions emerged. Jokowi was reluctant to use the word "COVID-19 lockdown" in his public speeches as a lockdown would concede that his political opponent Baswedan was right. Potentially worried about antagonizing Islamic leaders, Jokowi resisted calls for banning homecoming during the end of Ramadan (*mudik*) and instead elected for permit-based travel restrictions. By December 2020—in a cabinet reshuffle—Putranto was replaced by Budi Gunadi Sadikin, a former banker as the health minister, reflecting the Jokowi administration's perception of the crisis in economic terms.

By May 2021, as COVID-19 cases began to balloon in Indonesia, following the rapid spread of the Delta variant. Jokowi followed his earlier example of resisting calls for a nationwide lockdown. Instead, he advocated for mass vaccination as a technical fix to end the pandemic. But low vaccine supplies and vaccination rates could not keep pace with the rapid spread of the variant. To his credit, Jokowi was rapid in sourcing vaccine supplies from China in January 2021. But Indonesia was also a victim of the global vaccine divide and struggled to procure more effective vaccines such as those produced by Pfizer or Moderna.[129] By June 2021, instead of a nationwide lockdown, he called for

Emergency Enforcement of Community Activity Restrictions (PPKM Darurat) in Java and Bali to prevent community transmission. Again, he avoided the use of the word lockdown to prevent the dampening of overseas investors' confidence in Indonesia.

Jokowi realized that the pandemic provided the perfect opportunity to realize his dream of a powerful and highly developed Indonesia. This was evident in his constant exhortations to Indonesians to take on new productive mindsets and habits and not be downcast by the pandemic. In May 2020, as a part of the country's new normal campaign, Jokowi mobilized some 340,000 Indonesian military (TNI) and police personnel—reminiscent of the New Order era and a deepening of the securitization process— across the archipelago to enforce the government's COVID-19 protocols.[130] Apart from the TNI, the Jokowi administration has enlisted the support of the BIN (Indonesian Intelligence Agency) for enforcing COVID-19 protocols. In his address to the nation on October 20, 2021, Jokowi compared the COVID-19 crisis to a fire. "If we can, we prevent it but if it happens there are many lessons that we can learn from it."[131] Furthermore, he drew a parallel between the pandemic [that killed over 100,000 Indonesians] and an economic recession to emphasize strengthening the resilience of the Indonesian economy, particularly the health infrastructure.

Even before the COVID-19 pandemic struck Indonesia, Indonesian healthcare was among the most under-resourced in Southeast Asia with an adverse health worker–to–population ratio and public health spending, estimated to be 3.1 percent (2012), lower than either the Philippines or Vietnam.[132] All this meant that the health system was unable to cope with the COVID-19 crisis that became evident in the sharp rise in COVID-19 cases in July 2021. This was true, particularly in Java. Hospitals on the island were pushed to the brink due to staffing shortages; and a shortage of the wonder drug remdesivir used to treat patients and a shortage of oxygen cylinders and beds forced patients to return home.

The history of public health helps contextualize Indonesia's economy-first approach to the COVID-19 crisis that was earlier evident during the Soekarno Era when the campaign against endemic diseases was implemented. During the 1950s, with a view to obtain international technical assistance in health, the government essentially downplayed the holistic approach to health and instead, adhered to a narrow program of disease eradication.[133] Since the first wave of COVID-19, the country's response to the pandemic has been skewed in favor of economic growth and less toward the population's health. Expectations of the Indonesian public from medical professionals to be more vigilant about their political role, as advocates of the poor—a legacy that was bequeathed by nationalist physicians such as Boentaran Martoatmodjo (Indonesia's first Minister of Health between August 19, 1945, and November 14, 1945)—continues with response to the COVID-19 pandemic.[134]

Notes

1 Johannes Leimena, "Ten Years Activities of the Ministry of Health: August 1945–August 1955," *Berita Kementerian Kesehatan* 5, no. 2 (1956): 5–12.
2 Johannes Leimena, *The Upbuilding of Public Health in Indonesia* (Jakarta: Pertjetakan Negara, 1950), 13.
3 See also Vivek Neelakantan, "Indonesianization of Social Medicine," *Lembaran Sejarah* 10, no. 1 (2013): 74–86.
4 Refer Vivek Neelakantan, *Science, Public Health and Nation-Building in Soekarno Era Indonesia* (Newcastle-upon-Tyne: Cambridge Scholars, 2017). See also Saki Murakami, "'Call for Doctors!' Uneven Medical Provision and Modernization of State Health Care During the Decolonization of Indonesia, 1930s-1950s," in *Cars, Conduits and Kampongs: The Modernization of the Indonesian City, 1920–1960*, eds. Freek Colombijn and Joost Cote (Brill: Leiden, 2014), 29–62. For an exception, refer Hans Pols, *Nurturing Indonesia: Medicine and Decolonisation in the Dutch East Indies* (Cambridge: Cambridge University Press, 2018). Although Pols' monograph transcends the colonial–postcolonial divide, the intersections between the Cold War and Indonesian medical history remain cursorily explored.
5 Januar Achmad, *Hollow Development: The Politics of Health in Soeharto's Indonesia* (Canberra: ANU Press, 1999).
6 See, for example, Eric Stein, "Vital Times: Power, Public Health and Memory in Rural Java" (PhD Thesis, University of Michigan, 2005).
7 For the appropriation of military metaphors by Indonesian physicians, refer to Vivek Neelakantan, "The Campaign Against the 'Big Four' Endemic Diseases and Indonesia's Engagement with the WHO During the Cold War 1950s," in *Public Health and National Reconstruction in Post-War Asia: International Influences, Local Transformations*, eds. Liping Bu and Ka-che Yip (Abingdon: Routledge, 2014), 154–74.
8 Anne Booth, "Government and Welfare in the New Republic: Indonesia in the 1950s," *Itinerario* 34, no. 1 (2010): 57–76. DOI: 10.1017/S0165115310000057.
9 Booth, "Government and Welfare," 62.
10 Leimena, "Ten Year Activities," 8.
11 Elizabeth Fee, Marcos Cueto and Theodore Brown, "At the Roots of the World Health Organization's Challenges: Politics and Regionalization," *American Journal of Public Health* 106, no. 11 (2016): 1912–17, https://doi.org/10.2105/ajph.2016.303480.
12 Ibid.
13 A summary of the speech in "DEFENSE and World Health," *Public Health Report* 65, no. 49 (1950): 1611–13.
14 Vivek Neelakantan, *Science, Public Health and Nation-Building in Soekarno-Era Indonesia* (Newcastle-Upon-Tyne: Cambridge Scholars, 2017), 68.
15 Neelakantan, *Science, Public Health and Nation-Building*, 68.
16 "Request by the United States of Indonesia for Inclusion in the South-East Asia Area: Supplementary Agenda Item 13.2," Third World Health Assembly A3/85, May 12, 1950, WHO Library, Geneva (WHOL).
17 Letter, "Ministry of Health, the Republic of the United States of Indonesia (Johannes Leimena) to Minister of Health, Republic of India (Raj Kumari Amrit Kaur)," March 9, 1950, *WHO First Generation Files* (WHO.1, 1945–1950), WHO Archives, Geneva (WHOA).
18 Johannes Leimena, "World Health and World Community," *The Ecumenical Review* 4 (1956): 407–9.
19 Johannes Leimena, *Kewarganegaraan Yang Bertanggung Jawab* (Jakarta: BPK Gunung Mulia, 1980), 73.

20 C.E.A. Winslow, *The Cost of Sickness and the Price of Health* (Geneva: WHO, 1951), 75–77.

21 Leimena, *Public Health in Indonesia: Problems and Planning* (Djakarta: GCT van Dorp and Co., 1956).

22 Ibid.

23 Johannes Leimena, *Some Aspects of Health Protection to Local Areas in Indonesia* (Geneva: publisher unknown, 1953).

24 The estimated cost for setting up auxiliary hospitals attached to health centers at the subdistrict level in 1954 was approximately 1 million rupiah (equivalent to US$131,000 at 1952 exchange rates). During the early 1950s, with a view toward achieving a favorable ratio of one hospital bed per 1000 population, the central government spent 44 million rupiah (equivalent to US$5.7 million) in constructing new hospitals and upgrading existing ones. The central government transferred the construction of new hospitals from the Ministry of Public Health to the Ministry of Public Works. But due to shortages of personnel, the construction of new hospitals was handed to private contractors. The expenses for construction or upgradation of hospitals were difficult to determine due to high inflation and stagnation of per capita income of average Indonesians. Refer Leimena, *Public Health in Indonesia*. For a wider understanding of the Indonesian state's shortcomings in raising peoples' living standards, see also Benjamin Higgins, "Indonesia's Development Plans and Problems," *Pacific Affairs* 29, no. 2 (1956): 107–25. http://www.jstor.org/stable/2752601?origin=JSTOR-pdf.
    Health financing during the Soekarno era was supported by two legal precedents: (a) the Constitution of 1945 that obliged the state to manage all sectors of the economy for the greatest benefit of the people and (b) the Basic Law on Health (1960) that guaranteed a minimum standard of health for all Indonesians. But the aspirational health law could not be implemented even toward the end of the Soekarno era due to hyperinflation and provincial rebellions, particularly in West Sumatra and South Sulawesi that continued to challenge the authority of Jakarta. The rank of civil servants ballooned from 145,000 toward the end of Dutch colonialism to 807,000 by 1960. At the time, civil servants were the only Indonesians with any kind of health insurance. For a nuanced understanding of health financing in postcolonial Indonesia, refer to Elizabeth Pisani, Maarten Olivier Kok and Kharisma Nugroho, "Indonesia's Road to Health Coverage: A Political Journey," *Health Policy and Planning* 32 (2017): 267–76, https://doi.org/10.1093/heapol/czw12.

25 Neelakantan, *Science, Public Health and Nation-Building*, 77.

26 Dewan Perwakilan Rakjat, "Rapat 88: Landjutan Pembitjaraan Rantjangan Undang Undangan Tentang Kesehatan," *Risalah Perundingan Dewan Perwakilan Rakjat*, June 20, 1951.

27 Neelakantan, *Science, Public Health and Nation-building*, 79.

28 Ibid., 54.

29 Ibid.

30 Dewan Perwakilan Rakjat, "Rapat 76: Undang Undang Tentang Penundjukan Rumah Sakit Partekulir Jang Merawat Orang Miskin dan Orang Jang Kurang Mampu," *Risalah Perundingan Dewan Perwakilan Rakjat*, May 22, 1953.

31 In Makale, South Sulawesi, the missionary hospital received a grant from the central government. But the provincial government of South Sulawesi was not enlisted in the management of the hospital.

32 Neelakantan, *Science, Public Health and Nation-Building*, 78.

33 Dewan Perwakilan Rakjat, "Rapat 19," *Risalah Perundingan Dewan Perwakilan Rakjat*, September 29, 1950.

34 Neelakantan, *Science, Public Health and Nation-Building*, 78.

35 Risalah Perundingan Dewan Perwakilan Rakjat, "Rapat 76."

36 Vivek Neelakantan, "The Campaign Against the Big Four," 160.
37 Soekarno, "Amanat Presiden Soekarno Pada Ulang Tahun Proklamasi Kemerde-kaan Indonesia, 17 Agustus 1955 di Djakarta," in *Dibawah Bendera Revolusi* (Dja-karta: Panitia Dibawah Bendera Revolusi, 1965), 148.
38 Soekarno, "Amanat Presiden Soekarno Pada Ulang Tahun Proklamasi Kemerde-kaan Indonesia, 17 Agustus 1959 di Djakarta," 228.
39 Neelakantan, "The Campaign Against the Big Four," 160.
40 Randall Packard, *Global Health: A History of Global Health: Interventions into the Lives of Other Peoples* (Cambridge: Cambridge University Press, 2018).
41 "Draft of Eisenhower's Speech," White House Correspondence General 1955(2), John Foster Dulles Papers Box 5, *White House Memorandum Series*, Dwight Eisen-hower Presidential Library.
42 Neelakantan, "The Campaign Against the Big Four Endemic Diseases," 161.
43 Ibid.
44 Kevin Fogg, "Indonesian Socialism of the 1950s: From Ideology to Rhetoric," *Third World Quarterly* 42, no. 3 (2020): 465–82, https://doi.org/10.1080/014 36597.2020.1794805.
45 For details regarding the U.S. pressure to slow down Indonesia's malaria eradica-tion program, refer Neelakantan, *Science, Public Health and Nation-Building*, 105.
46 Ibid.
47 Ibid.
48 Guy Pauker, "Political Doctrines and Political Practices in Southeast Asia," *Pacific Affairs* 35, no. 1 (1962): 3–10.
49 Ragna Boden, "Cold War Economics: Soviet Aid to Indonesia," *Journal of Cold War Studies* 10, no. 3 (2008): 110–28.
50 Ibid.
51 *Untuk Perdamaian dan Kesedjahteraan Rakjat* (Djakarta: Bagian Penerangan Besar URSS, 1960).
    D.D. Venediktov and V.I. Petrov, *Untuk Taraf Kesehatan jang Tertinggi* (Dja-karta: The Soviet Embassy, 1960).
52 Satrio and Mona Lohanda, "Perjuangan dan Pengabdian: Mosaik Kenangan Pro-fessor Dr Satrio, 1916-1986," *Penerbitan Sejarah Lisan* 3 (Jakarta: Arsip Nasional Republik Indonesia, 1986), Published Oral History Collection of Arsip Nasional Republik Indonesia.
53 Ibid.
54 Indonesia accounted for 20 percent of the world's tin output, 38 percent of the global production of natural rubber and the only source of crude petroleum in the Western Pacific. For specific details of U.S. strategic interests in Indonesia refer Correspondence, "The Acting Secretary of State for Far Eastern Affairs (Allison) to Mr. Robert Blum (Special Assistant to Asst. Admin for Program, ECA)," Decem-ber 31, 1951, Doc. 463, in *Foreign Relations of the United States, 1951, Asia and the Pacific* Volume 6, Part 1, eds. Paul Claussen, John Glennon, David Mabon, Neal Petersen and Carl Raether (Washington, DC: Government Printing Office, 1977), Department of State Office of the Historian Website. Accessed via https:// history.state.gov/historicaldocuments/frus1951v06p1/d463.
55 Herb Feith, *The Decline of Constitutional Democracy in Indonesia* (Singapore: Equinox Publishing, 2007), xii.
56 "Special Report on Indonesia," File NSC 5518: Policy on Indonesia (1)," NSC Series Policy Papers Sub Series Box 16, *White House Office of the Special Assistant for National Security Affairs Records, 1952–61*, Dwight Eisenhower Presidential Library.
57 For details, refer to Neelakantan, *Science, Public Health and Nation-Building*, 166–70.

58 "Text of President Soekarno's Address to the Congress, 1956," Folder Title "Soekarno's Speeches," Folder 1, Box 292, *Henry Kissinger Papers Part II, Series I: Early Career and Harvard University*, Manuscripts and Archives, Yale University. Accessed via: http://yul-fi-prd1.library.yale.internal/catalog/digcoll:560301.

59 Terence Hull and Valerie Hull, "Dari Keluarga Berencana ke Pelayanan Reproduksi: Sebuah Riwayat Singkat," in *Masyarakat, Kependudukan dan Kebijakan di Indonesia*, Terence Hull and Valerie Hull ed. (Jakarta: Equinox, 2006), 3.

60 Neelakantan, *Science, Public Health and Nation-Building*, 56.

61 Ibid.

62 Soekarno, "Amanat Presiden Soekarno," 147.

63 Neelakantan, *Science, Public Health and Nation-Building*, 57.

64 Hull and Hull, "Dari Keluarga Berencana," 14.

65 Ibid.

66 Departemen Kesehatan Republik Indonesia, *Sejarah Kesehatan Nasional Republik Indonesia*, Vol 2. (Jakarta: DEPKES, 1978), 144.

67 Eric Stein, "Hygiene and Decolonization: The Rockefeller Foundation and Indonesian Nationalism,1933–58," in *Science, Public Health and the State in Modern Asia*, in Liping Bu, Darwin Stapleton and Ka-che Yip ed. (Abingdon: Routledge, 2012), 51-70.

68 Hilmar Farid, "Rethinking the Legacies of Bandung," *Inter-Asia Cultural Studies* 17, no. 1 (2016): 12–18, https://doi.org/10.1080/14649373.2016.1133387.

69 Farid, "Rethinking the Legacies of Bandung," 16.

70 "Speech by President Soekarno at the Afro-Asian Congress of Pediatrics in Istana Negara, Djakarta," August 15, 1964. *Monash Collections Online*. Accessed via https://repository.monash.edu/items/show/12492.

71 "Defiance of US Repeated," *The New York Times*, May 4, 1964, https://www.nytimes.com/1964/05/04/archives/defiance-of-u-s-repeated.html.

72 A.M. Taylor, "Soekarno: First United Nations Dropout," *International Journal* 20, no. 2 (1965): 206–13, https://doi.org/10.2307/40199519.

73 Adrian Vickers, *A History of Modern Indonesia, Second Edition* (Cambridge: Cambridge University Press, 2013), 158.

74 Ibid.

75 Ibid.

76 Neelakantan, *Science, Public Health and Nation-Building*, 196.

77 Vickers, "A *History of Modern Indonesia*, 148.

78 Pols, *Nurturing Indonesia*, 216.

79 See, for example, "Gestapu: Gerakan September Tiga Puluh, G-30-S, September 30th Movement," in *Historical Dictionary of Indonesia*, by Robert Cribb and Audrey Kahin (Lanham, MD: Scarecrow Press Inc., 2004), 159–60.

80 Ibid.

81 Firman Lubis recounts his participation in these movements as a medical student at Universitas Indonesia. See Firman Lubis, *Jakarta 1960-An: Kenangan Semasa Mahasiswa* (Jakarta: Masup, 2008), 265.

82 See, for example, "Telegram from the Embassy in Indonesia to the Department of State: Subject Meeting with Soeharto," July 7, 1967, Doc. 236, in *Foreign Relations of the United States, 1964-68: Indonesia; Malaysia-Singapore; Philippines* Volume 26, ed. Edward Keefer (Washington, DC: US Government Printing Office, 2000), Department of State Office of the Historian Website. Accessed via: https://history.state.gov/historicaldocuments/frus1964-68v26.

83 For details, refer to Graeme Thompson and Richard C. Manning, "The World Bank in Indonesia," *Bulletin of Indonesian Economic Studies* 10, no. 2 (1974): 56–82. https://doi.org/10.1080/00074917412331332479.

84 Brad Simpson, "Indonesia's 'Accelerated Modernization' and the Global Discourse of Development, 1960-75," *Diplomatic History* 33, no. 3 (2009): 467–86. http://www.jstor.org/stable/44214022.

85 Simpson, "Indonesia's 'Accelerated Modernization,'" 475.

86 Simpson, "Indonesia's Accelerated Modernization," 477.

87 "Soeharto: The Giant of Modern Indonesia Who Left a Legacy of Violence and Corruption," *The Conversation*, August 21, 2021, https://theconversation.com/soeharto-the-giant-of-modern-indonesia-who-left-a-legacy-of-violence-and-corruption-164411.

88 Pols, *Nurturing Indonesia*, 218.

89 DEPKES, *Sejarah Kesehatan Nasional Indonesia* Volume 3 (Jakarta: DEPKES, 1980), 13.

90 Viktor Nikijulow and Erlita Rachman, eds., *Sang Upuleru: Mengenang 100 Tahun Professor Dokter Gerrit Siwabessy, 1914–2014* (Jakarta: Gramedia, 2014).

91 Socrates Litsios, "The Long and Difficult Road to Alma Ata: A Personal Reflection," *International Journal of Health Services* 32, no. 4 (2002): 709–32, https://doi.org/10.2190/rp8c-l5ub-4raf-nrh2.

92 Socrates Litsios, "On the World Health Organization's Neglect of the Role of Medical Doctors in Its Conception and Practice of Primary Healthcare," *International Journal of Health Services* 49, no. 3 (2019): 642–57, https://doi.org/10.1177%2F0020731419840914.

93 Gunawan Nugroho, "Indonesia: Starting from Scratch," *World Health: Magazine of the World Health Organization* (April 1975): 26–30.

94 Ibid. For a parallel with China, refer Xun Zhou, *The People's Health: Health Interventions and Delivery in Mao's China, 1949–83* (Montreal: McGill-Queen's University Press, 2020), 12. By the late 1970s, the "Chinese approach to health" came to hold out the promise of a true alternative to the crumbling, single disease-centered "vertical" health care program advocated by the U.S. or the centralized health care structure of the Soviet Union.
    Nugroho, "Starting from Scratch."

95 Ibid.

96 Ibid.

97 Januar Achmad, *Hollow Development: The Politics of Health in Soeharto's Indonesia* (Canberra: ANU, 1999), 5.

98 The World Bank, "Indonesia Health Sector Overview," February 20, 1979, Document 2379-ID, *World Bank East Asia and Pacific Regional Office*, http://documents.worldbank.org/curated/en/393801468268184401/Indonesia-Health-sector-overview.

99 Vivek Neelakantan, "Eradicating Smallpox in Indonesia: The Archipelagic Challenge," *Health and History* 12, no. 1 (2010): 61–87. PubMed ID: 20973337.

100 Neelakantan, "Eradicating Smallpox," 74.

101 Terence Hull, "Formative Years of Family Planning in Indonesia," in *The Global Family Planning Revolution: Three Decades of Population Policies and Programs* in Warren Robinson and John Ross ed. (Washington, DC: The World Bank, 2007), 235–57.

102 Hull, "Formative Years," 238.

103 Ibid., 239.

104 Donald Warwick, "The Indonesian Family Planning Program: Government Influence and Client Choice," *Population and Development Review* 12, no. 3 (1986): 453–90, http://www.jstor.org/stable/1973219.

105 Warwick, "The Indonesian Family Planning Program," 467.

106 Ibid.

107 Terence Hull, Valerie Hull and Masri Singarimbun, "Indonesia's Family Planning Challenge: Success and Failure," *Population Bulletin* 32, no. 6 (1977): 4–45.

108 Ibid.

109 Hull, Hull and Singarimbun, "Indonesia's Family Planning Challenge," 10.

110 Ibid.

111 Hull, Hull and Singarimbun, "Indonesia's Family Planning Challenge," 3.

112 Pols, *Nurturing Indonesia*, 225.
113 Steve Ferzacca, "Mediations of Health and Development of a Nation: Late Soeharto, Late Modernity," in *Liberalizing, Feminizing and Popularizing Health Communication in Asia*, Liew Kai Khiun, ed. (Farnham, MA: Ashgate, 2010), 15–42.
114 Dewi Fortuna Anwar, "Fall of Suharto: Understanding the Politics of the Global," in *Southeast Asian Responses to Globalization: Restructuring Governance and Deepening Democracy*, Francis Loh Kok Wah and Joakim Öjendal, ed. (Copenhagen: NIAS, 2010), 201–32.
115 For specific details refer Neelakantan, *Science, Public Health and Nation-Building*, 206.
116 Leimena, "Ten Year Activities."
117 Pramoedya Ananta Toer and Sumit Mandal, "My Kampung," *Indonesia* 61 (April 1996): 25–31, http://www.jstor.org/stable/3351361.
118 See "Undang Undang Republik Indonesia Nomor 9 Tahun 1960 Tentang Pokok Pokok Kesehatan" (Djakarta:Kementerian Penerangan, 1960).
119 Achmad, *Hollow Development*, 140–41.
120 Ibid., 171.
121 See Pisani, Kok and Nugroho, "Indonesia's Role to Universal Coverage."
122 Celia Lowe, "Viral Sovereignty Security and Mistrust as Measures of Future Health in the Indonesian H5N1 Influenza Outbreak," *Medical Anthropology Theory* 6, no. 3 (2019): 109–32, https://doi.org/10.17157/mat.6..3.662.
123 Lowe, "Viral Sovereignty," 117.
124 Ibid.
125 News Desk, "Indonesia Well Prepared to Handle the Coronavirus Outbreak," *The Jakarta Post* January 29, 2020, https://www.thejakartapost.com/news/2020/01/29/indonesia-well-prepared-to-handle-coronavirus-outbreak-who.html.
126 Tim Lindsey and Tim Mann, "Indonesia Was in Denial Over Coronavirus. Now It May Be Facing Looming Disaster," *The Jakarta Post*, April 9, 2020, https://www.thejakartapost.com/academia/2020/04/09/indonesia-was-in-denial-over-coronavirus-now-it-may-be-facing-a-looming-disaster.html.
127 A. Ibrahim Al Muttaqi, "The Omnishambles of COVID-19 Response in Indonesia," *The Habibie Center Insights* (13/23 March 2020), https://www.habibiecenter.or.id/img/publication/4210e17bd7d6d8d29223ec3791f1412e.pdf.
128 Ibid.
129 Charlotte Setijadi, "The Pandemic as a Political Opportunity: Jokowi's Indonesia in the Time of COVID-19," *Bulletin of Indonesian Economic Studies* 57, no. 3 (2020): 297–320, https://doi.org/10.1080/00074918.2021.2004342.
130 Greg Fealy, "Jokowi in the Covid-19 Era: Repressive Pluralism, Dynasticism and the Overbearing State," *Bulletin of Indonesian Economic Studies* 56, no. 3 (2020): 301–23, https://doi.org/10.1080/00074918.2020.1846482.
131 Ikbal Tawakal, "Jokowi Analogikan Krisis, Resesi, Hingga Pandemi Covid-19 Itu Seperti Api," *Pikiran Rakyat*, October 20, 2021, https://www.pikiran-rakyat.com/nasional/pr-012839025/jokowi-analogikan-krisis-resesi-hingga-pandemi-covid-19-itu-seperti-api.
132 See, for example, Y. Mahendranatha, S. Listyadewi, L. Trisnantoro, P. Soewondo and T. Marthias et al., "The Republic of Indonesia Health System Review," *Health System in Transition* 7, no. 1 (2017), The World Health Organization Regional Office for Southeast Asia, New Delhi, https://www.apps.who.int/iris/handle/10665/254716.
133 See also Ka-che Yip and Liping Bu, "Introduction: National Health, International Interests," in *Public Health and National Reconstruction in Post-War Asia: International Influences: Local Transformations*, 1–12.
134 See also Neelakantan, "The Campaign Against the Big Four," 155.

Index

Pages in *italics* refer to figures and pages followed by "n" refer to notes. Personal names followed by (RF) indicated Rockefeller Foundation staff.

For Product Safety Concerns and Information please contact our EU
representative GPSR@taylorandfrancis.com
Taylor & Francis Verlag GmbH, Kaufingerstraße 24, 80331 München, Germany